Butterworths International Medical Reviews

Otolaryngology 1

Otology

Butterworths International Medical Reviews

Otolaryngology 1

Next volume in this Series

Plastic Reconstruction

Butterworths
International
Medical
Reviews

Otolaryngology 1

Otology

Edited by
Alan G. Gibb, MB ChB, DLO, FRCS
Head of Department of Otolaryngology
University of Dundee; and
Senior Consultant Otolaryngologist
Ninewells Hospital
Dundee, UK

and

Mansfield F. W. Smith, MD
Clinical Associate Professor of Surgery
Division of Otolaryngology – Head and Neck Surgery
Stanford University Medical Center, Stanford
California; and
Ear Medical Clinic of Santa Clara Valley
San Jose
California, USA

Butterworth Scientific
London Boston Durban
Singapore Sydney Toronto Wellington

First published 1982

©Butterworth & Co. (Publishers) Ltd. 1982

British Library Cataloguing in Publication Data

Otology. –
(Butterworths international medical reviews:
Otolaryngology ISSN 0260-0102; 1)
1: Otolaryngology
I. Gibb, Alan G.   II. Smith, Mansfield F. W.
617.8   RF121

ISBN 0-407-02318-6

Photoset by Butterworths Litho Preparation Department
Printed and bound in England by Robert Hartnoll Ltd, Bodmin, Cornwall

Preface

The otologist of the present day has available a wealth of books, journals and other publications to ease his task of keeping abreast of the speciality. However, the abundance of published materal merely aggravates rather than solves his problem so that it has become increasingly important for the busy otologist to be selective in his choice of reading material. In this Medical Review Series outstanding instructional sessions presented at International Congresses have been chosen as the basis of the text. The contributors have been selected carefully and are internationally recognized as experts in their particular subjects. These instructional sessions all had a wide appeal at their respective symposia, yet the details of these presentations have not hitherto been published. We felt, therefore, that those who attended the sessions and found them valuable, and many others who were unable to attend, would welcome having the contents available in published form. Our selection aims at a balanced review of the main developments in otology so that other instructional sessions, equally in demand, have been excluded for this reason and because of space limitations.

Chapters on pathophysiology form an important part of the text as we feel that progress in otology must go hand in hand with a sound understanding of the normal functioning of the ear and the pathological processes to which it is subject. These sections are of great importance in relation to recent developments in cochlear implantation, in the treatment of tinnitus and fluctuant hearing loss and in the management of facial paralysis. The giddy patient still constitutes a diagnostic challenge, and despite the availability of sophisticated labyrinthine tests, the onus continues to rest on the otologist to accurately interpret the results in relation to each specific clinical problem. As is pointed out in the text, history taking still remains of paramount importance in the diagnosis of all problems of dysequilibrium.

The present status of middle ear surgery is reviewed by various experts who outline their personal techniques and give the reasons for their choice. Arguments continue regarding the merits of open and closed techniques in mastoid surgery but it is of more than passing interest to note that some of the earlier enthusiasm for closed mastoid surgery, which swept the specialty like a tidal wave, is now on the wane. Opinions also differ regarding the use and value of prosthetic materials in middle ear reconstruction, and while some of the earlier materials have already been discarded in favour of human tissues, we must wait for a further period before passing judgement on later prosthetic developments, especially the use of ceramic materials.

A review of the current status of stapedectomy in otosclerosis was considered timely, especially since, with the passage of time, the evaluation of long-term results is now possible. There is now general agreement that a sound tissue seal of the oval window is desirable to prevent fistula development. Prosthetic materials are still widely used to replace the stapes superstructure but time may yet show that human materials are preferable especially in the younger age group.

In the audiological field we have included an instructional session on electrical response audiometry, where recent developments have greatly assisted in the diagnosis of eighth nerve tumours and have also made possible the objective measurement of pure tone hearing thresholds in young children and in cases of suspected non-organic hearing loss. The latter condition is now assuming increasing importance because of the great rise in the number of industrial claims following altered legislation. Furthermore the incidence of ototoxicity appears to be on the increase as more potent drugs are discovered and introduced. In affected cases litigation frequently follows and the exclusion of non-organic hearing loss is mandatory.

The Review Series is designed to provide a balanced view of the present state of otolaryngology and to keep the specialist in touch with important developments. Subsequent editions are planned to cover other fields in the specialty.

Our thanks are due to all our contributors for co-operating so expeditiously in the production of this edition. We would also express our gratitude to our publishers, Butterworths, for their valuable assistance in our editorial tasks.

List of Contributors

John C. Ballantyne, FRCS, Hon FRCS(I)
Consultant ENT Surgeon, Royal Free Hospital, London, UK; Consultant ENT
Surgeon, King Edward VII Hospital for Officers, London, UK

Derald E. Brackmann, MD
Clinical Professor of Otolaryngology, University of Southern California; Otologic
Medical Group Inc., and House Ear Institute, Los Angeles, California, USA

R. Ross A. Coles, MB, FRCP (Edin.), DLO
Deputy Director and Co-ordinator of Clinical Studies, MRC Institute of Hearing
Research, Nottingham, UK

Roger L. Crumley, MD
Associate Clinical Professor, Department of Otolaryngology – Head and Neck
Surgery, University of California, San Francisco, California, USA

Manuel Don, PhD
Director, Auditory Research Laboratory, House Ear Institute, Los Angeles,
California, USA

E. F. Evans, BSc, MB, ChB, PhD
Professor of Auditory Physiology and Head of Department of Communication and
Neuroscience, University of Keele, Staffordshire, UK

Ronald E. Gristwood, MB, ChB, FRCS (Edin.), FRACS
Lecturer-in-Charge of Otorhinolaryngology, University of Adelaide; Chairman,
Department of Otorhinolaryngology and Senior Visiting Otorhinolaryngologist,
Royal Adelaide Hospital, Adelaide, Australia

Jack van Doren Hough, MD
Clinical Professor of Otorhinolaryngology – Head and Neck Surgery, University of Oklahoma Health Sciences Center, Oklahoma; Otologic Medical Clinic Inc., Oklahoma City, Oklahoma, USA

Howard P. House, MD
Clinical Professor of Otolaryngology, University of Southern California School of Medicine; President, House Ear Institute; Otologic Medical Group Inc., Los Angeles, California, USA

Brian F. McCabe, MD
Professor and Head, Department of Otolaryngology – Head and Neck Surgery, University of Iowa Hospitals and Clinics, Iowa City, Iowa, USA

Tauno Palva, MD
Professor of Otolaryngology and Head, Department of Otolaryngology, University of Helsinki, Helsinki, Finland

Dietrich Plester, MD
Professor of Otolaryngology; Director of Ear, Nose and Throat Clinic, Eberhard-Karls-University, Tübingen, West Germany

Weldon A. Selters, PhD
Audiologist, Otologic Medical Group Inc., Los Angeles, California, USA

James L. Sheehy, MD
Clinical Professor of Otolaryngology, University of Southern California School of Medicine; Director, Audio-visual Department, House Ear Institute; Otologic Medical Group Inc., Los Angeles, California, USA

Mansfield F. W. Smith, MD
Clinical Associate Professor of Surgery, Division of Otolaryngology – Head and Neck Surgery, Stanford University Medical Center, Stanford, California; Ear Medical Clinic of Santa Clara Valley, San Jose, California, USA

G. D. L. Smyth, DSc, MCh (Hons), MD, FRCS, DLO
Consultant Surgeon, Eye and Ear Clinic, Royal Victoria Hospital, Belfast, UK

Contents

Part 1
Tympanomastoid problems

1
Tympanomastoid disease
Gordon D. L. Smyth

INTRODUCTION

Although disease of the tubotympanic cleft takes many forms, including primary and secondary neoplasia, collagen disorders, congenital abnormalities and specific infections such as syphilis and tuberculosis, in the majority of cases it is primarily the result of inflammation, usually associated with bacterial infection.

This chapter is concerned only with the latter, and will discuss the aetiology of chronic otitis media, its clinical presentations and their underlying pathology in order to provide a basis for the understanding of the varied manifestations of this frequently incapacitating and persistently common world health problem. Chronic otitis media is no respecter of social status or geographical location and, although much progress in its treatment has been made during the past two decades, many obstacles still remain to be overcome. Not only does highly sophisticated and expensive equipment need to be much more widely available but – in order to be effective – this has to be accompanied by a greater understanding of the basic nature of the disease, which is possible only by the continued free dissemination of knowledge, particularly that learnt in the recent past.

Although the introduction of the operating microscope heralded a new era in otology, early methods of microsurgery of necessity involved much trial and error with skills and materials. Painstaking clinical research has provided much information not only about successful techniques but also about causes of failure, and it is hoped that this will provide a basis for continued advances in the future.

One of the aims of this chapter is to draw attention to the results of some well-intentioned, but eventually unsuccessful procedures, the disadvantages of which are not yet widely recognized, and to suggest ways in which the outlook for patients with chronic otitis media might be improved.

AETIOLOGY

Although it may well be true that in the past chronic otitis media was frequently the consequence of acute suppurative otitis media, present-day experience does not

3

support such a clear-cut relationship between acute and chronic infections of the middle ear (McCabe, 1977). Although in developed communities necrotizing otitis media is occasionally observed, its incidence is so markedly disproportionate to the numbers of ears presenting *de novo* with various abnormalities of the tympanic membrane as to call into question the importance of such a cause-and-effect relationship. The theory advocated by aurists of the Vienna era of otology, namely that squamous ingrowth through a pre-existing perforation was the predominant cause of cholesteatoma, is, in the light of prolonged study of such ears, also no longer tenable.

The differences in clinical presentation of the various types of chronic inflammatory disease of the middle ear and mastoid air cells have led to the evolution of a number of separate theories as to their causation. However, repeated observations and accurate recording over long periods of time have led to support the view that all of the varied forms of chronic suppurative otitis media derive from one single root cause, namely unresolved middle ear effusion (Smyth, 1980). There is considerable evidence that such effusions contain enzymes capable of destroying both the ossicular chain, especially the particularly vulnerable, relatively avascular lenticular process of the incus, and – more importantly – the fibrous elements of the tympanic membrane (Abramson, 1969). Not only does such damage tend to perpetuate the effusion by reducing the 'drumhead's' elasticity, thus impairing the membrane's ability to aspirate air into the middle ear while the Eustachian tube is opened by swallowing, but – and more importantly – it creates in the membrane an area of diminished vitality which renders it liable to necrosis during any subsequent inflammatory process, and to a permanent perforation.

Should the tympanic membrane lose its inherent elasticity, coexistent perpetual negative pressure will lead either to total collapse of the tympanic membrane, resulting in atelectasia, or to partial collapse, usually postero-superiorly (Austin, 1977b), where the enzymatic action of fluid entrapped in the confined space of the crowded ossicular anatomy and associated mucosal folds leads to the commonly observed retraction pocket. Although loss of elasticity cannot explain retraction of Shrapnell's membrane (which lacks elastic fibres), again, negative pressure may well be an important aetiological factor. Here the pressure deficiency, which is confined to the epitympanum and parts distal to it, is caused by obstruction of the isthmi anticus and posticus (Smyth, 1975).

An alternative theory, based more on animal studies than clinical observation, to explain the development of cholesteatoma from Shrapnell's membrane and also, possibly, from the postero-superior quadrant of the pars tensa, postulates that proliferation of the basal cells of the squamous epithelium of the tympanic membrane results in an inward growth of surface tissue which later becomes canalized to form an invasive pouch (Ruedi, 1958). It is proposed that the stimulus for such a process derives either from elements contained in middle ear effusion or from superficial irritants (Steinbach, 1978). A third, less widely supported, explanation for the development of cholesteatoma is based on experiments which demonstrate that changes in gaseous environment and substrate on tissue cultures can affect the histological characteristics of primitive cells (Sade, 1977). As a consequence, instead of cuboidal epithelium, islands of keratinizing squamous epithelium (originating in the epitympanum or postero-superior areas of the mesotympanum) could develop and, growing laterally around the ossicles, lead eventually to necrosis of the tympanic membrane.

In both types of cholesteatoma – postero-superior and epitympanic – the subsequent events are similar and have a common mechanism. Because growth of squamous epithelium is a continual process, and because its direction is now abnormal, i.e. inwards, there is a perpetual risk of keratin accumulation and the eventual development of a cholesteatoma. As has been well described over the years, this condition, otherwise termed keratoma or epidermoid, is one of 'skin in the wrong place', but pathologically it is much more than that. Associated with this keratinizing squamous epithelium is a substratum of granulation tissue which, by virtue of its enzymatic action and an accompanying shift in pH, causes demineralization and osteolysis leading to further extension of the cholesteatomatous process; as is well known, this may result in severe hearing loss accompanied by the threat of labyrinthine and intracranial complications.

Because such lesions interfere with normal aeration, chronic inflammatory changes develop in mucosa and bone of the mastoid air cell system, leading to the formation of granulation tissue and a combination of bone destruction and osteoneogenesis (Friedmann, 1957).

Atelectasia and cholesteatoma are obviously the most dangerous complications of unresolved middle ear effusion because of their potential threat to functional capacity and life; however, another serious condition, not involving ingrowth of keratinizing squamous epithelium and its inherent risks, also commonly presents. This is chronic granulomatous middle ear disease in its fully developed form, 'cholesterol granuloma'. In this, the pathological findings are similar with regard to mucosal and osseous involvement. However, there is no keratinizing epithelium and the potentially lethal complications of cholesteatoma, which appear in some way to be related to the presence of a foreign body, namely keratin, are lacking.

Although both conditions appear to share a common origin, their outcome may vary considerably, mainly because of differences in subsequent development (Smyth, 1980). Whereas cholesteatoma occurs following structural changes in the intact tympanic membrane due to enzymatic digestion, cholesterol granuloma is the result of secondary inflammation, which, because of prior loss of tympanic membrane vitality in that ear, leads to a permanent defect. This creates a potential for recurrent contamination from the nasopharynx (because of altered aerodynamics) or from the external auditory meatus. If the tubotympanic cleft's powers of recovery become inadequate, the pathological state will persist indefinitely. The concept of Politzer (1902), which invokes modern theories of tissue contact inhibition (Sade, 1977) and the restraining effect of the annulus fibrosis on epithelial ingrowth, probably still holds true as an explanation for the absence of keratinizing epithelium in such cases.

Hence, in summary, it is postulated that all of the varieties of chronic middle ear disease stem from unresolved middle ear effusion. In the presence of lowered host resistance or exceptional bacterial or viral virulence, permanent perforation, with or without the development of cholesterol granuloma, occurs. Although the view that less active inflammatory processes may lead to atelectasia is attractive, in the absence of contrary evidence, the possibility of persistent effusion acting as a stimulus for either basal cell proliferation or metaplasia of primitive middle ear epithelium cannot be ruled out. Whatever the exact mechanism, an association between middle ear effusion and all forms of chronic otitis media appears highly likely.

TREATMENT

The options of treatment for most forms of human disease range between control and cure – a precept which certainly applies to the therapy of chronic otitis media, depending upon the facilities available and the need of the patient. Although eradication of dangerous disease must remain the premier surgical aim at all social levels, in more developed communities the restoration of function assumes some importance and has attracted increasing attention in recent years.

Nevertheless, otologists are still most concerned with the basic problem of converting the chronically diseased into a permanently stable ear which is free from any threat of intracranial complications and the inconvenience of persistent drainage. If aural function can be improved, or even restored, this is certainly a desirable bonus but definitely of secondary importance.

In other words, surgical treatment may be necessary for reasons of survival or general improvement of health, or, in more sophisticated and wealthy societies, it may be related to other needs commensurate with the patient's life style. The precise aims of surgical treatment must be clearly understood by both patient and surgeon. Such an understanding depends on the surgeon's accurate evaluation of the patient's disability, his explanation of the problem and his potential to solve it, coupled with the patient's capacity to understand that explanation.

Preoperative considerations

The patient should be informed, both verbally and by letter, about the general nature of the operation proposed and the likely outcome. Personal experience and knowledge gained from routine follow-up and careful record maintenance should enable the surgeon to predict the outcome with reasonable accuracy.

The choice of surgical technique is determined by the type and extent of the disease process, and ranges from myringoplasty, with or without repair of the ossicular chain, to operations in which the mastoid air cells are also opened in order to reach diseased tissue not accessible by a purely transcanal route.

The decision to operate is based on the nature of the pathological state and on the need for, and possibility of, functional improvement. Cholesteatomatous disease practically always requires eradication and, particularly in young persons, this should be done as soon as possible after diagnosis in order to prevent the development of ossicular lesions which will prejudice the ultimate auditory status.

Patients who present an anaesthetic risk (usually due to serious circulatory disease) may be better managed by frequent suction clearance of cholesteatoma, which can be performed under the operating microscope as an outpatient procedure.

The persistently or recurrently draining ear will almost always require some form of operative treatment in order to eliminate unacceptable symptoms and improve function.

Although surgical intervention for eradication of chronic disease is justified and necessary in almost all cases, the indications for treatment of hearing impairment are by no means so clear-cut, and it must be emphasized that careful judgement is always necessary in this respect. Firstly, the cochlear reserve must be such that correction of a conduction hearing loss will result in a useful auditory gain for the patient. If postoperatively the patient still relies on his contralateral ear, the operation will have achieved little. The importance of this aspect of preoperative selection is highlighted by the not inconsiderable incidence of unsuccessful results due to tympanic membrane graft failure, inefficient ossicular reconstruction and sensorineural defects arising from surgical trauma (Smyth, 1977).

It is frequently stated that normal Eustachian tube function is an essential prerequisite for a successful outcome in tympanoplasty. Although there can be no argument that a normally functioning tube is the ideal, opinions about how best to evaluate its function vary. It can be argued that such preoperative evaluations are superfluous and may even be dangerous if they lead to a decision against operation. Malfunction at the diagnostic interview may be due to tubal obstruction by an anteriorly collapsed tympanic membrane, polyps and granulation tissue, oedema of the tubal mucosa, or toxic effects on the cilia – all of which can be expected to be overcome by surgical restoration of the tympanum and subsequent healing of the mucosa. Radiological studies are also considered by some surgeons to be a necessary part of the preoperative work-up. Certainly they will provide information regarding the degree of mastoid sclerosis, but this should not in any important way influence a decision regarding the need for, or type of, operation. It has been proposed that high quality tomography has value in detecting labyrinthine fistula, but it could be argued that this is an unnecessary procedure because, in practice, *all* ears with cholesteatomatous disease should be regarded as potentially complicated by fistula until shown otherwise during the operation. This can be done by carefully opening the cholesteatoma sac to allow palpation and inspection of the contours of the lateral and posterior semicircular canals; if a fistula is detected, the steps of the operation are then ordered appropriately. The reliance on radiography rather than routine microscopic inspection in the outpatient clinic in the diagnosis of cholesteatoma will inevitably result in many dangerous situations.

Because bacteria frequently participate in chronic otitis media, their role in the disease (whose fundamental mechanism is enzymatic) has possibly been overestimated. It is certainly true that aerobes, and on occasion anaerobes, can be cultured from most discharging ears, but their role is secondary and should not be allowed to diminish the importance attached to the removal of keratinizing epithelium and irreversibly diseased tissue, such as inflamed mucosa, granulations and abnormal bone, which creates an anatomical basis for the restoration of healthy epithelial and mucosal structures. Although the suppression of infectious organisms would be a desirable adjunct to excisional surgery, in many instances the currently available antibacterial and antiviral agents are inappropriate to the organisms most frequently encountered. Although supportive statistical evidence of their value is so far lacking, many surgeons use broad-spectrum antibiotics for prophylactic purposes, especially when homologous or biocompatible materials are used. The best justification for routine culture and sensitivity determinations of preoperative secretion would appear to be that valuable information is available should unexpected postoperative complications occur (personal communication).

Surgical techniques

The eradication of disease and the prevention of its recurrence

Maintenance or restoration of the normal anatomical state has been the goal of most recent innovations based on microsurgical techniques. In particular, the problem of avoiding an open mastoidectomy cavity and of preserving the dimensions of the meso- and epitympanum has preoccupied many surgeons during the past two decades. Unfortunately, much of what promised to be a transformation in terms of better long-term results has proved disappointing, and techniques such as combined approach or intact canal wall tympanoplasty (Jansen, 1963; *Figure 1.1*) have, in the light of experience, too often failed to fulfil the hopes of their protagonists. Not only has it been shown by several planned studies of two-stage

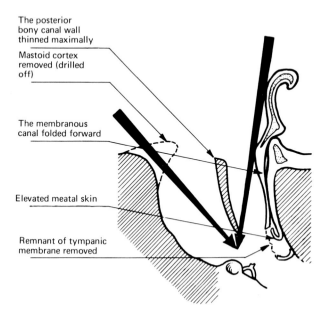

The posterior
bony canal wall
thinned maximally

Mastoid cortex
removed (drilled
off)

The membranous
canal folded forward

Elevated meatal skin

Remnant of tympanic
membrane removed

Figure 1.1 A combination of the transcanal and transmastoid routes enables the surgeon to expose mesotympanic disease without removing the osseous canal wall, i.e. combined approach tympanoplasty. (From Jansen, 1963, courtesy of the Editor and Publishers, *Laryngoscope, St Louis*, **73**, 1288–1294)

procedures that there is an unexpectedly high incidence of failure to totally remove keratinizing squamous epithelium at the first stage (when the surgeon was certain he had done so), but also that there is a formidable incidence of postoperative retraction pocket formation, i.e. a recurrence of the original disease, in all forms of combined middle ear and mastoid disease when the canal wall is preserved (Austin, 1977a; Wright, 1977; Smyth, 1981). Throughout the early clinical 'experiment' with canal wall up procedures, there were surgeons who, recognizing the technical difficulties of the procedure and the limitations which were frequently imposed on visualization by the constricted anatomy, argued that a better alternative, particularly for achieving a safe ear, was the removal of the canal wall to provide better access to the epitympanum and the posterior areas of the mesotympanum (Palva, Karma and Palva, 1977). This was combined with immediate obliteration of the mastoid area with a postaurally based soft tissue plug to avoid postoperative cavity problems (*Figures 1.2–1.4*). This procedure certainly led to excellent healing results; nevertheless, the incidence of failure to totally eradicate keratinizing epithelium from the epi- and mesotympanum has been shown at re-exploration operations to be no less than with canal-preserving techniques (Smyth, 1977).

Hence we are left with the unavoidable conclusion that, for the safety of the patient, 'closed' operations must always be staged and repeated until the surgeon can detect no more evidence of residual disease in any part of the tubotympanic cleft.

Apart from the advantage of rapid and continued healing of the mastoid bowl, it has been claimed that 'closed' techniques are the best means of improving function because there is less anatomical distortion. Again, unfortunately, this claim has not

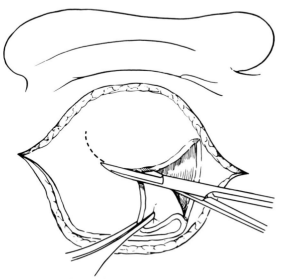

Figure 1.2 The pedicled soft tissue graft is carefully tailored so that it matches as closely as possible the dimensions of the mastoid bowl. The graft is divided into two segments so that an elongated L-shaped strip is formed from its superior and posterior parts in order to enable the graft to reach the epitympanum and fill the mastoidectomy cavity. (From Smyth, 1980, courtesy of the Publishers, *Chronic Ear Disease*)

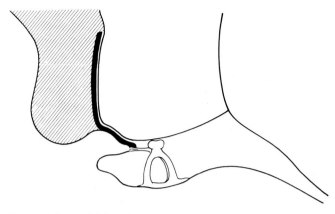

Figure 1.3 Rapid healing of the meatus and the prevention of retraction pockets are achieved by separating the remnants of meatal skin from the obliterating flap with a carefully positioned layer of autologous temporalis fascia or preserved dura mater

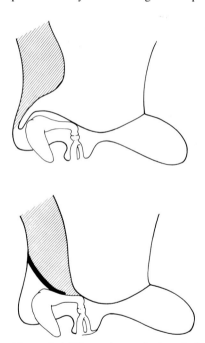

Figure 1.4 When the ossicular chain is preserved, the tendency for retractions to form superiorly and medially (top) can be prevented by supporting the Palva graft with a film of cartilage (bottom). (From Smyth, 1980, courtesy of the Publishers, *Chronic Ear Disease*)

been confirmed. In fact, using the same methods of tympanic membrane and ossicular chain repair, it has been shown that the presence or absence of the osseous canal wall exerts no significant influence on final function (Smyth and Hassard, 1981). If an operation comprising canal wall down with mastoid obliteration and tympanic reconstruction has any advantage over the combined approach technique, this is the low incidence of eventual retraction pocket formation in the former (Smyth, 1981). Otherwise there certainly does not appear to be much to differentiate them, apart from the greater technical difficulties of combined approach tympanoplasty. Both procedures must be carried out in two or more stages and both produce similar alterations in auditory capacity.

Because a reliable once-only operation obviously would be preferable to both patient and surgeon, a re-evaluation of the surgical treatment of chronic ear disease is now in progress. To some extent this has become necessary because of attitudes created by the 'magic' of microsurgery and also, of necessity, because of the time required to allow a long-term and balanced viewpoint. The introduction of the operating microscope appears to have led to the assumption that all previous methods could be discarded in favour of newer and, by implication, better techniques. The error of this concept is now becoming increasingly apparent and a more moderate view is emerging which concedes the undeniable value of micro-surgical technique, especially in tympanic reconstruction, but also recognizes the

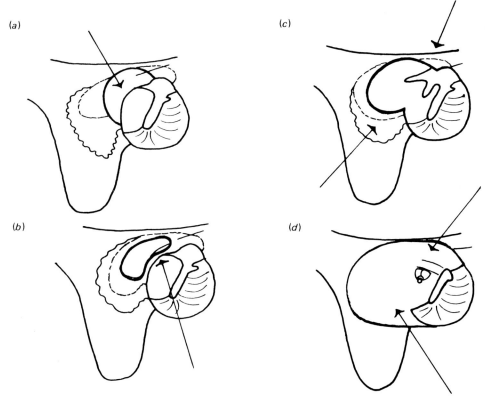

(a)

(c)

(b)

(d)

Figure 1.5 (*a*) Initially bone removal is performed directly towards the epitympanum and aditus. (*b*) Having opened the aditus, the extent of the cholesteatoma is assessed, and with the ossicular chain in view the 'bridge' (arrow) and further bone removal is carried out as required. (*c*) Although exposure of keratinizing epithelium does not always require extensive removal of bone, in order to achieve a stable mastoidectomy cavity, overhanging bone in the region of the 'facial ridge' and the posterior root of the zygoma (arrows) is essential. (*d*) Having removed all overhanging areas of bone as indicated, a symmetrical cavity is created with a potential for rapid epithelialization

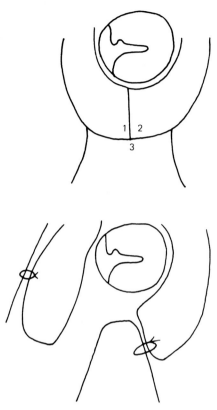

Figure 1.6 Following the elevation of a tympanomeatal flap, the posterior meatal and conchal skin is divided into three segments (1–3) and a crescent of conchal cartilage (4 × 2.5 mm) is excised (top). Following the completion of mastoidectomy these flaps are secured as indicated (bottom). The superior flap is sutured to the lower margin of the temporalis muscle and the middle and inferior flaps brought together in the floor of the cavity

advantages of more traditional methods. Hence there is now a new school of thought which advocates a combination of the almost century-old technique of modified radical mastoidectomy with modern developments in repair of the tympanic membrane and ossicular defects in order to offer the patient a once-only procedure which would give him a safe, healed ear with a reasonable chance of functional improvement and the possibility of a minor secondary procedure if a further attempt for auditory gain is desirable and justified.

The operating microscope and hypotensive anaesthesia are obviously indispensable for this combined new procedure. The surgical technique, no less demanding than those of the earlier microsurgical otological operations, requires expert clearance of all irreversibly diseased soft tissue and bone from each area of the tubotympanic cleft, concluding with a symmetrical open mastoid bowl (*Figure 1.5*). The traditional Stacke and Korner flaps, with excision of conchal cartilage to ensure a wide meatal orifice (*Figure 1.6*), are essential adjuncts to healing (Schuknecht, Chasin and Kurkjian, 1966). Subsequent self-contamination of the cavity is prevented by reconstruction of the tympanic membrane, and, whenever possible, auditory function is improved by repair of any ossicular chain defects. The arguments in support of this revitalized 'open' technique are several – those against relatively few.

In favour are:

(1) appropriate skin flaps result in rapid cavity healing
(2) residual disease in the mastoid bowl and epitympanum will be obvious and can be easily treated on an outpatient basis
(3) recurrent disease is entirely avoided
(4) useful presurgical hearing is maintained and in some cases even improved. This benefit applies to ears in which an intact chain or a natural myringo-stapediopexy can be maintained – both frequently impossible with the combined approach method.

Arguments against this new 'open' technique are: (1) routine postoperative visits will remain a necessity for inspection and cleansing of the mastoid bowl. However, because such visits are equally necessary with 'closed' techniques in order to detect complications, this is not a very potent criticism. (2) The incidence of residual cholesteatoma in the mesotympanum cannot be expected to be less than with 'closed' techniques. However, so far, this has not been shown to be as dangerous as it undoubtedly is when it occurs in the epitympanum and mastoid segment, and must therefore remain an accepted cost of closing the tympanum in order to avoid reinfection of the cavity and to facilitate functional improvement.

Although, at first glance, such a return towards the fundamental methods of the Politzer era of otology may appear retrogressive, the results argue otherwise. A once-only method is obviously infinitely preferable to a staged one. The hearing results are no worse and, indeed, may well be significantly better, especially when the decision to operate is made early rather than late.

None of the above should be taken to encourage technical shortcuts or a lowering of standards in dexterity – far from it. The proposed system, developed from the experience which has preceded it, demands the utmost in expertise and judgement. Insufficient knowledge of temporal bone anatomy, the varieties of the pathological processes, and unskilled removal of diseased tissue (without a wide meatoplasty and the creation of appropriate skin flaps), will still lead to the same unsatisfactory results which have previously retarded progress in the treatment of chronic mastoid disease.

Tympanic reconstruction

As already stated, permanent eradication of irreversible disease is the basis for success in tympanoplasty. This, of necessity, depends upon the surgeon's ability to prevent subsequent problems which arise from failure of the mesotympanum to heal – repair of tympanic membrane defects is vital. Fortunately such repair carries a high degree of success with all of the most commonly used methods. Although opinions still vary with regard to materials and their site of placement, a better than 90% success rate can be expected with most techniques.

This particular aspect of treating chronic otitis media presents no great difficulty when the extent of the disease requires mastoidectomy of whatever type, largely because access to the perforation is unrestricted. However, when disease is limited to the mesotympanum and the lesion comprises a tympanic membrane defect with or without discontinuity of the ossicular chain, its solution may be less easily achieved. This particularly applies to defects involving the anterior part of the membrane, to which access is frequently impeded by a prominence of the anterior osseous canal wall. The key to success with this problem is the achievement of a clear view of the anterior sulcus, either by removing the anterior overhang directly through the meatal orifice, often by an endaural incision which is time-comsuming, or by approaching the problem area obliquely through postaural and transmeatal skin incisions. In practice, the latter is usually simpler and avoids the problem of 'blunting' which can occur when the anterior meatal skin is temporarily displaced, as in the former technique.

The postaural route permits excision of the epithelial rim of the defect, minimal displacement of the annulus fibrosis and application of the graft material to the anterior wall of the mesotympanum, where it is supported by Gelfoam. As with all myringoplasty techniques, placement of the graft material is assisted by raising a preliminary tympanomeatal flap, which also gives access to lesions of the ossicular chain. Autologous temporalis fascia is the generally preferred material for repair of the tympanic membrane, but advocates of preserved homologous dura mater claim a similar take rate (except in ears with combined active suppuration and total defects, in which the results are significantly less successful) and better ease of handling (Smyth, Kerr and Goodey, 1971). An earlier vogue for the tympanic membrane homograft appears to be waning, possibly because of lack of supply, cost factors and some unsatisfactory results.

Although there has been considerable interest in biocompatible materials for the repair of ossicular chain defects, most of the available statistics concerning their efficiency and tolerance by the ear do not suggest that their use will constitute a major breakthrough in otological surgery (Sheehy, 1978a; Smyth and Hassard, 1982). However, work in this field continues and it may be that developments with ceramic materials and tissue adhesive will lead to improvements over current standard techniques. Of these, natural autologous and homologous materials such as ossicular bone and nasal and tragal cartilage have been shown to provide predictable long-term results and good acceptance by the host; however, success rates continue to be inversely proportional to the extent of the lesion (another potent argument for operating early rather than late). At the same time, the effectiveness of these natural materials cannot escape the influence of factors such as the eventual health and aeration of the middle ear space and the compliance of the reconstructed tympanic membrane. In short, a successful auditory result depends on more than the nature of the prosthetic material itself; and if it is correct – as appears reasonable – that in ears where adherence of a columella to the stapes footplate is required, the possibility of host–tissue ingrowth is a necessary characteristic for the material used, then ossicular bone is very possibly the most suitable graft material so far available. It is porous (because of its Haversian canal system), has the ability to become revitalized and is virtually never extruded; there thus seems much in favour of continued efforts to perfect the techniques already in use with ossicular bone grafts, provided adequate safeguards are taken to avoid the risks of transmitting disease from donor to host when the material is homologous. There is increasing support for the concept of performing ossicular reconstruction as a secondary procedure. Staging the operation is an attractive concept in that the transmission system is constructed after mucosal healing and ventilation of the middle ear has occurred and when, in addition, the position of the grafted tympanic membrane is stable. Staging would appear to be particularly appropriate in patients with bilateral disease in order to improve the chances of attaining useful function in at least one ear.

Special problems

Labyrinthine fistula

In the past, mastoid surgery in the presence of this complication of cholesteatoma has led to many functionless ears, complicated by disequilibrium and tinnitus. Opinions as to its management are not yet agreed and all methods carry some risk of catastrophe.

As stated previously, awareness of the possible existence of fistula in *all* such ears, regardless of whether the fistula test is negative or not, greatly assists in a successful outcome.

With 'closed' techniques the layer of keratinizing epithelium overlying the labyrinthine defect should be preserved intact until the final stage of the operation. Some surgeons will then carefully dissect this layer and immediately replace it with a piece of temporalis fascia (Palva, Kärjä and Palva, 1971), while others prefer to leave the fistula undisturbed for six months before cleaning it (Law, Smyth and Kerr, 1975; Sheehy, 1978b). Those who favour the latter method claim a lower incidence of postoperative sensorineural hearing loss. It is worth noting that fistulae of the lateral semicircular canal are frequently accompanied by dehiscence of the facial nerve.

Tympanosclerosis

This pathological variant of chronic otitis media has assumed increased importance in parallel with advances in ear surgery for functional restoration.

Plaques of tympanosclerotic material causing immobility of the ossicular chain must be removed or bypassed if sound energy is to be adequately transmitted to the cochlea. Removal, especially from the oval window, carries an indisputable risk of hair cell damage due to hydraulic effects or fistulization of the footplate and is one of the main causes of sensorineural hearing loss as a complication of tympanoplasty (Smyth, 1972). There are surgeons who now believe that if such ears require operation the procedure should be limited to only that which is necessary for the eradication of suppurative or cholesteatomatous processes and to tympanic membrane repair and that no attempt should be made to restore ossicular, and in particular stapedial, mobility, certainly never at the first operation. Many would then prefer to improve auditory function in such an ear by means of amplification with a hearing aid, which in many instances gives an acceptable result and certainly carries no risk of irreversible inner ear dysfunction.

The 'only hearing ear'

There will always be patients who, having lost all useful function in one ear because of infectious labyrinthitis or previous operations, later require surgical treatment to avoid serious inflammatory complications in the other ear. Such a situation imposes very definite limitations on what can and should be done. Any technique which might endanger the cochlea must be scrupulously avoided. Although this may not prevent repair of the tympanic membrane in ears where discontinuity of the ossicular chain has already occurred, it certainly proscribes any attempt at ossicular reconstruction. This conclusion is based on a recognized, though admittedly small, incidence of sensorineural hearing loss even in apparently straightforward myringoplasty (Smyth, 1977). The best management would appear to be marsupialization by means of 'open' mastoidectomy, combined with an ample meatoplasty to facilitate healing and future cleansing, and to allow the fitting of a hearing aid should this become necessary.

CONCLUSIONS

Following the birth of the modern era of otological surgery, there has inevitably been a period of trial and error in order to determine to what extent and in which way microsurgical techniques could best be put to the service of the hard of hearing.

In the realm of tympanomastoid disease, after 20 years' experience, it has now become apparent that some of the methods which were developed in the hope of restoring normal function and permanent freedom from disease are less successful than had been hoped. Nevertheless, some useful lessons have been learned. Possibly the most important of these is that there was much merit in traditional techniques, upon which new expertise can now be built with much more satisfactory results than were previously possible.

These lessons can no longer be ignored and persistence with methods now proven misconceived can certainly not be justified. There is still very much to be said in favour of 'open' techniques, provided they are carried out with the highest possible degree of skill and appropriate use of recent technological advances in magnification, instrumentation and anaesthesia. Further advances will depend upon a better recognition of the need to understand which factors are primarily responsible for the occurrence of chronic otitis media and how the effects of persistence of these can be controlled or eliminated.

References

Abramson, M. (1969) Collagenolytic activity in middle ear cholesteatoma. *Annals of Otology, Rhinology and Laryngology*, **78**, 112–124

Austin, D. F. (1977a) On the function of the mastoid. *Otolaryngological Clinics of North America*, **10**, 541–547

Austin, D. F. (1977b) The significance of the retraction pocket in the treatment of cholesteatoma. In *Cholesteatoma* (First International Conference), pp. 379–383. Birmingham, Alabama: Aesculapius

Friedmann, I. (1957) The pathology of otitis media with particular reference to bone changes. *Journal of Laryngology and Otology*, **71**, 313–319

Jansen, C. (1963) Cartilage tympanoplasty. *Laryngoscope*, 1288–1302

Law, K. P., Smyth, G. D. L. and Kerr, A. G. (1975) Fistulae of the labyrinth treated by staged combined approach tympanoplasty. *Journal of Laryngology and Otology*, **89**, 471–478

McCabe, B. F. (1977) The etiology of chronic otitis media. *Clinical Otolaryngology*, **3**, 243–248

Palva, T., Kärjä, J. and Palva, A. (1971) Opening of the labyrinth during chronic ear surgery. *Archives of Otolaryngology*, **91**, 75–78

Palva, T., Karma, P. and Palva, A. (1977) Cholesteatoma surgery: canal wall down and mastoid obliteration. In *Cholesteatoma* (First International Conference), pp. 363–367. Birmingham, Alabama: Aesculapius

Politzer, A. (1902) In *Diseases of the Ear*, 4th Edn., edited by M. J. Ballin and C. L. Heller. London: Ballière, Tindall & Cox

Ruedi, L. (1958) Cholesteatosis of the attic. *Journal of Laryngology and Otology*, **73**, 593–609

Sade, J. (1977) Pathogenesis of attic cholesteatoma: the metaplastic theory. In *Cholesteatoma* (First International Conference), pp. 212–232. Birmingham, Alabama: Aesculapius

Schuknecht, H. F., Chasin, W. and Kurkjian, J. (1966) *Stereoscopic Atlas of Mastoid-Tympanoplastic Surgery*. St Louis, Mo: C. V. Mosby Co.

Sheehy, J. L. (1978a) TORPs and PORPs in tympanoplasty. *Clinical Otolaryngology*, **3**, 451–454

Sheehy, J. L. (1978b) Management of the labyrinthine fistula. *Clinical Otolaryngology*, **3**, 405–414

Smyth, G. D. L. (1972) Tympanosclerosis. *Journal of Laryngology and Otology*, **86**, 9–14

Smyth, G. D. L. (1975) Surgical treatment of chronic otitis media: problem cases. *Transactions of the Pacific Coast Oto-ophthalmological Society*, **56**, 195–202

Smyth, G. D. L. (1977) Sensorineural hearing loss in chronic ear surgery. *Annals of Otology, Rhinology and Laryngology*, **86**, 3–8

Smyth, G. D. L. (1980) *Chronic Ear Disease*. New York: Churchill Livingstone

Smyth, G. D. L. (1982) What do we find at second operations? In *Cholesteatoma and Mastoid Surgery*, edited by J. Sade. Amsterdam; Kuyler (1982)

Smyth, G. D. L. and Hassard, T. H. (1981) The evolution of policies in the surgical treatment of acquired cholesteatoma of the tubotympanic cleft. *Journal of Laryngology and Otology*, **95**, 767–773

Smyth, G. D. L. and Hassard, T. H. (1982) Malleus to oval window techniques: TORPs and PORPs. In *Proceedings of the Sixth Shambaugh Workshop*. Strode Publications (in press)

Smyth, G. D. L., Kerr, A. G. and Goodey, R. J. (1971) Current thoughts on combined approach tympanoplasty. IV. Results and complications. *Journal of Laryngology and Otology*, **85**, 1021–1029

Steinbach, E. (1978) Tierexperimentelle Untersuchungen zur Enzeugung von Cholesteatomen. *Laryngologie, Rhinologie, Otologie (Stuttgart)*, **57**, 724–733

Wright, W. K. (1977) A concept for the management of otic cholesteatomas. In *Cholesteatoma* (First International Conference), pp. 374–378. Birmingham, Alabama: Aesculapius

2
Obliteration of the mastoid cavity and reconstruction of the canal wall

Tauno Palva

INTRODUCTION

Up to the beginning of the 1950s the creation of an open operation cavity was the accepted policy in the surgical treatment of chronic osteitic ear disease. A modified radical operation meant preserving the ossicles and the remains of the tympanic membrane, whereas the radical operation included removal of the malleus and incus together with the tympanic membrane as far as the annulus. The goal of surgery was to create a safe open mastoid bowl, and by introduction of the modified radical operation an attempt was made to preserve useful preoperative hearing. The ideal outcome was a skin-lined open cavity with a wide meatus allowing easy inspection and removal of accumulating keratin debris and cerumen. The meatal skin grew inwards into the open cavity, covering also the medial tympanic walls in cases with radical surgery.

It was generally acknowledged that a proportion of the open cavities became badly infected, and some ears were worse after surgery than they had been preoperatively. In some ears the cavity was filled with granulation tissue and there was copious discharge from the ear. These ears were certainly not safe. At that time, large-scale antibiotic treatment and microsurgical techniques were just being introduced. In our own early studies (Palva and Pulkkinen, 1960) the frequency of continuously discharging cavities was close to 10%, and 20% were occasionally moist, but other series from that period (Beales, 1959) reported a rate of infected open cavities as high as 60%.

I started reconstructive middle ear surgery in the early 1950s, using ossicles and skin. Operative methods improved as microsurgical techniques came into use, and the tympanoplastic methods, developed by Wullstein and Zöllner, spread rapidly. However, as fascial tissue began to come into use and, before long, replaced skin in middle ear surgery, the scene was ready for a major change in surgical policy. On the one hand, Myers and Schlosser (1960) advocated preservation of the ear canal with the 'anterior-posterior' technique, combining mastoidectomy with transmeatal work through an ear speculum. This procedure, in a modified form, was also advocated by Jansen (1963) and has become known as the 'canal wall up' procedure or 'combined approach tympanoplasty'. On the other hand, both Guilford (1961) and Palva (1963) emphasized the inadequacy of the canal wall up technique for removal of cholesteatomatous epithelium, and the canal wall down procedure was therefore recommended for all ears in which the cholesteatoma could not be removed by a limited endaural atticotomy. We recommended obliteration of the mastoid cavity with postauricular tissues, Guilford using an inferiorly or superiorly based flap, whereas my flap was based meatally.

In 1959 I started using cavity obliteration in cholesteatoma surgery and for many years the meatally based musculo-periosteal flap was the only material I used. The osseous meatus was not reconstructed. When the flap was tailored to fit the expected cavity (as estimated on the basis of the radiograph), all ears with small, and most ears with medium-sized cavities later presented an ear canal only slightly wider than normal (Ojala, 1979). If large mastoid bowls were created, however, about 30% of the ears showed distinct cavitation. These were, in reality, small open cavities requiring regular removal of wax and keratin.

Realizing that additional tissue had to be employed when obliterating large mastoid cavities, I first used inorganic heterologous bone posterior to the musculo-periosteal flap. Later, bone pâté from the patient's own cortical bone was used to fill all posterior crevices of the open cavity. In addition, the ear canal wall was reinforced by periosteum-containing bone chips from the mastoid tip and lyophilized dura (Palva, 1973; Palva and Mäkinen, 1979).

Studies of temporal bones obtained at autopsy several years after surgery, and histological examination of musculo-periosteal flaps deliberately excised during revision surgery, showed that the muscle tissue in these flaps remained intact for years (Palva *et al.*, 1975). The postauricular branches of the facial nerve supplying the flaps were demonstrable in the excised flaps. The blood supply of both the superior and the inferior parts of the flap was not endangered during the formation of the flap, provided that the flap was made sufficiently large from the start. Thus, the flap was not subject to atrophy; yet if used alone, it could not possibly fill an extensive cavity but retracted posteriorly leaving a cavity-like ear canal.

SURGICAL TECHNIQUE

If the patient has a narrow ear canal, a Körner-type meatoplasty with extensive resection of conchal cartilage is made at the start of the operation (*Figure 2.1a*). In normal-sized ear canals relaxing incisions without cartilage resection can be made at points corresponding to 11 and 7 o'clock (right ear). No such incisions are required if the ear canal is large.

For formation of the musculo-periosteal flap, a curved skin incision is made about 2 cm away from the postauricular fold. The skin is first undermined posteriorly and then anteriorly to outline the area of the soft-tissue flap. As elastic fibres in all connective tissue tend to shrink, the flap should be made slightly broader and longer than the cavity estimate based on the radiograph. Incisions are made down to the bone superiorly, posteriorly and inferiorly and the flap is then dissected towards the anterior broad pedicle. Periosteum is not included in the tip of the flap, but as soon as dissection proceeds to the posterior limit of the sigmoid sinus, the posterior incision is deepened to the bone. Anteriorly, dissection is continued until the flap is attached at its base only at the level of the meatal bone (*Figure 2.1b*).

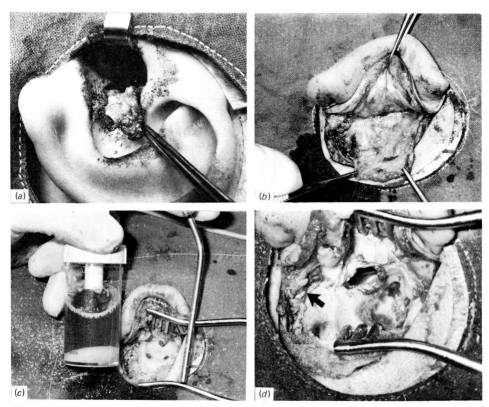

Figure 2.1 Preliminary steps for obliteration surgery. (*a*) In a narrow ear canal a meatal skin flap is raised and a suitable amount of conchal cartilage resected. (*b*) The meatally based musculo-periosteal flap is dissected. (*c*) Bone pâté is collected. (*d*) Ear canal skin is cut 2 mm inside the bony meatus. The arrow marks the area where the periosteum-containing bone chips have been collected

Bone pâté is collected by drilling the healthy cortical bone under continuous irrigation (*Figure 2.1c*). If a very large cavity must be made, material should also be collected from the bone over the temporal dura. The bone pâté is stored in ampicillin solution, or in some other non-ototoxic antibiotic solution, until used. Bone chips with attached periosteum are removed from the mastoid tip (*Figure 2.1d*) with a thin chisel and stored in the same way. The fascial graft is removed at this stage; if fascia is not available because of previous surgery, Cialit-stored dura is employed. I prefer to store the fascia under wet gauze to keep it soft until it is used.

The bone work in the mastoid is done thoroughly. Exposure and removal of disease from the sigmoid and middle fossa lamina generally marks the end of the bone work, but occasionally granulation-filled air cells are found up to the dura itself. In these cases it is advisable to expose the dura only in the diseased areas. It is rarely necessary today to resect a large area of dural lamina. If the dura is kept intact, no sequelae occur and obliteration of the cavity eliminates all risks of brain herniation should a dural tear or weakening have taken place.

In ears which have already been subjected to open cavity surgery and in which revision is undertaken either because of persistent suppuration or because of cholesteatomatous disease, special care must be taken to avoid damage to the sigmoid sinus and temporal dura and arachnoid. Both these structures may have been exposed and the cavity skin may now be intimately attached to the underlying tissue. Separation along the sigmoid wall must be made under the operating microscope with a sharp canal-wall elevator or a knife. Opening the sinus can then be avoided and all squamous epithelium removed. Should a rupture occur, the area need only be covered with Oxygel cottonoid and fascia. This will later be pressed in place by the obliterating material. In order to separate cavity skin from dura it may be necessary to deepen the resection in some areas to include three quarters of the dural layer. If dura must be removed in its full thickness and the arachnoid exposed, the area should be covered with fascia and muscle during the obliteration phase. There is no risk of brain herniation into the cavity if the obliteration is done properly.

When the mastoid bone work is completed, the dural and sigmoid laminae appear glistening white. Trautmann's triangle contains white bone and healthy vessels. The mastoid tip is empty down to the sternomastoid muscle, and the three semicircular canals can be distinguished. There is no risk that squamous epithelium is left anywhere in the cavity, which is now ready for obliteration. Removal of the posterior canal wall and creation of the swing doors greatly facilitates epitympanic and tympanic work (*Figure 2.2*). The incus and head of the malleus have to be removed in ears in which squamous epithelium grows on the medial surfaces of the ossicles. All bone covering the epitympanum must be drilled away so that one can inspect the whole laminar bone from the lateral surface medially to the area of the geniculate ganglion. Cholesteatoma frequently sends short offshoots into the bone and removal of only the main mass of squamous epithelium is certain to result in residual disease. It is advisable to use a large diamond drill and continuous irrigation to ensure faultless surgery on the laminar surfaces. The caudal edge of the excised bridge must be removed down to the level of the ear canal along the facial nerve canal. The pyramidal process and the bony canal containing stapedius tendon are then exposed, if need be, and the skin of the lower ear canal, together with the annulus and the remnant of the tympanic membrane, shifted anteriorly. Bone in this area often contains granulations which may contain papillary projections of squamous epithelium, revealed only by the microscope.

Surgery on the middle ear proper should proceed in a certain order (*Figure 2.3*). Cholesteatomatous mucosa is removed first from the promontory, the hypotympanum and the Eustachian tube, while the round and especially the oval window areas are cleaned out last. Similarly, if a horizontal semicircular canal fistula is present,

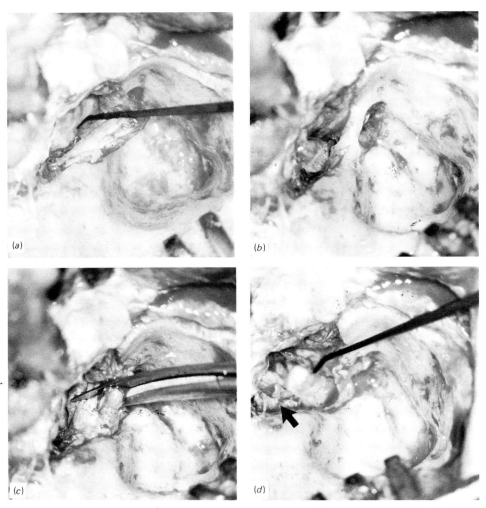

Figure 2.2 Creation of swing-door plasty of the canal skin (Palva, Palva and Kärjä, 1969). This technique greatly facilitates tympanic dissection and repair. (*a*) Posterior canal skin under the elevator. Swelling is produced by local injection of anaesthetic at the beginning of surgery. (*b*) Canal skin dissected forward with elevator. (*c*) Swing doors are made by cutting the skin down to the tympanic membrane perforation. (*d*) Lower swing door has been elevated (arrow) while the upper swing door is being raised with the elevator

this is cleaned as the last step. This operative order ensures cessation of all bleeding, and, as all major areas of infected tissue have been removed, the oval window (or fistula) can be cleaned under ideal conditions. Gelatin sponge soaked in ampicillin solution is frequently applied to the area while the work continues. Squamous epithelium in the oval window area can generally be removed without much difficulty. Sometimes squamous epithelium encircles the crura so intimately that the crura must be cut with delicate, curved neurosurgical scissors. This must be done with a very steady hand in order not to dislocate the footplate. The use of the argon laser has facilitated this phase of surgery enormously, as all suspected tissue in the oval window can be evaporated without gross movements.

The cleaning of a horizontal canal fistula can be safely undertaken under adequate magnification and illumination. The main point to remember is never to apply suction to the fistula. It should be protected with wet Gelfoam, soaked in ampicillin, while the membrane is lifted off with a broad-tipped thin canal-wall elevator. We have had no complications in planned removal of squamous epithelium. On the other hand, if one accidentally enters a fistula or the vestibule through the window, the ear may become deaf.

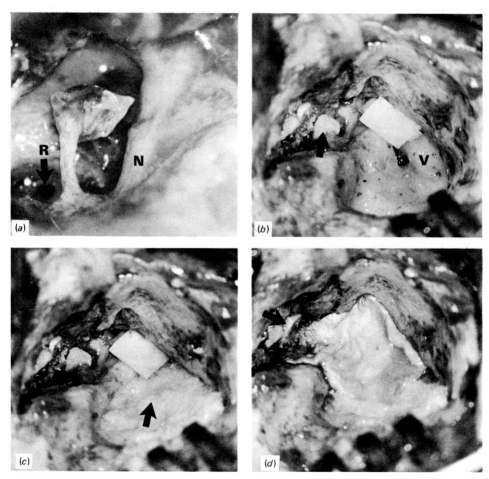

Figure 2.3 Tympanic reconstruction and initial steps for obliteration. (*a*) Last remnant of cholesteatoma around stapes head and crura. R = round window; N = facial nerve. (*b*) Cortical bone columella (arrow) on stapes head surrounded by pieces of gelatin sponge. Aditus ad antrum area is raised with lyophilized dura. V = vertical semicircular canal. (*c*) Bone pâté (arrow) has been pressed into the posterior cavity. (*d*) Anterior part of the temporal fascia is brought over the columella and under the tympanic membrane remnant (arrow) while the larger part lies temporarily on the bone pâté

The round window niche is often filled with a plug of swollen mucosa. I always remove it because (a) squamous epithelium may grow there unnoticed, and (b) the tissue may contain plenty of large secretory glands capable of functioning for a long time. There is seldom any risk of damaging the window membrane. Should a perforation occur, the membrane must be covered with a piece of fascia and the suction tip kept away from the area.

Reconstruction of the tympanic cavity should not be started until the surgeon is certain that he has removed all squamous epithelium medial to the tympanic membrane remnant. It should be borne in mind that migrating squamous epithelium may cover large areas of the medial surface of the tympanic membrane and extend to the promontory without producing clinically manifest cholesteatoma.

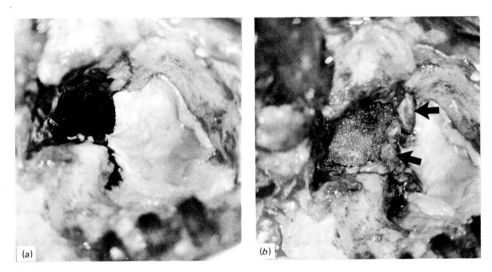

Figure 2.4 Primary steps in ear canal reconstruction. (*a*) A patch of cigarette paper soaked in a 0.5% solution of gentian violet fits snugly against the repaired tympanic membrane. (*b*) The swing doors have been taken back to their original position (arrows) and the lower half of the ear canal is filled with pieces of Merocel otowick or small gauze strips

Similarly, the advancing front of squamous epithelium may lie several millimetres beyond the keratin accumulation, which under the operating microscope appears to be the limit of the cholesteatoma. Poor results in terms of a high rate of residual disease are obviously due to a failure to understand the clinical behaviour of squamous epithelium. This can only be achieved by taking several biopsies from the tympanum and comparing histopathological findings with clinical appearance as recorded in the operative notes.

I employ thin strips of lyophilized dura to cover all bare surfaces, including those of the Eustachian tube, and perform the ossicular reconstruction with auto- or homologous ossicles or cortical bone. The tympanic membrane is reconstructed with underlaid temporal fascia. In cases of a total defect the fascia is placed anteriorly on the ear canal bone. The posterior portion of the new drumhead is raised with full-thickness lyophilized dura or bone chips. Small gauze strips are gently placed on top of the repaired tympanic membrane, which has first been covered with cigarette paper soaked in gentian violet (*Figure 2.4*).

As a preparation for obliteration of the cavity, the ear canal is filled with gentamicin (Garamycin) Vaseline tamponade (*Figure 2.5a*). The major part of fascia is then lifted up to cover the posterior surface of the canal skin from the epitympanum up to the level of the mastoid bone. The epitympanum is filled with strips of lyophilized dura (*Figure 2.5b*) and with periosteum-containing bone chips to make the posterior canal wall straight at the level of the facial nerve. Bone pâté

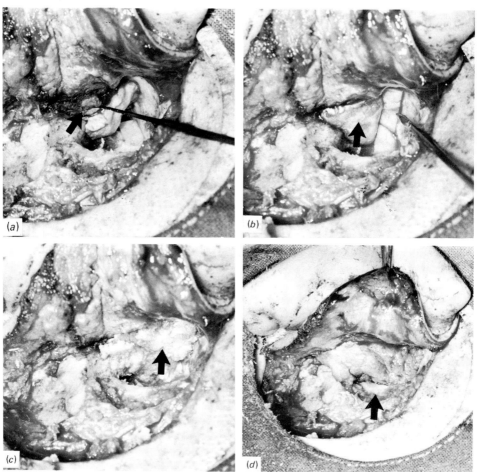

Figure 2.5 Final steps in obliteration. (*a*) The black elevator adjusts a gauze tamponade (arrow) brought through the ear canal to fill its upper part and to support the meatal skin flap in the correct position. (*b*) The remaining fascia (arrow) is lifted posterior to the meatal skin and the epitympanum is filled with strips of lyophilized dura (forceps point). (*c*) The soft ear canal wall is fortified with bone chips cemented in place with bone pâté (arrow). (*d*) The musculo-periosteal flap fills the remaining cavity. Arrow points to the lateral part of the sinus plate

is then pressed tightly into Trautmann's triangle and into the main cavity (*Figure 2.5c*). Depending upon the size of the cavity, the remaining space will be filled with the flap, which may now be turned in (*Figure 2.5d*). If there is still empty space, lyophilized dura, bone chips and bone pâté may be added until the filling is adequate. The final result should be a normal-sized ear canal with a tympanic cavity of normal height.

RESULTS AND DISCUSSION

Between 1964 and 1971 we used only the musculo-periosteal flap for obliteration. Follow-up examinations (on average 8.7 years after surgery) revealed that cavitation of the medial part of the ear canal had occurred in those ears in which the operation cavity had been extensive (Ojala, 1979). The normal ear canal volume of 0.8 ml had increased to 1.5 (sometimes even 2.5) ml in these ears, and both surface keratin and cerumen had started to accumulate because migration out of the ear was disturbed. This necessitated regular cleansing, usually at least once a year, and contributed to occasional infection of the ear canal. Nevertheless, in a series of 750 cases, the frequency of discharging ears at the time of follow-up (8.7 years) was only 3.1%, and in all these cases conservative treatment was effective. These findings prompted me to introduce the changes described above for improved obliteration and meatoplasty (Palva, 1973). Our present policy is to perform meatoplasty, under local anaesthesia, 1 year after surgery if cavitation associated with disturbance in cerumen and keratin transport is observed.

Our surgical team has devoted much time and effort to the study of squamous epithelium in the tympanic cavity, and it appears that we have removed suspicious epithelium much more thoroughly than many others. Our rate of recurrent cholesteatoma was 4.7% in ears evaluated on average 8.7 years after surgery (Ojala, 1979), while the 12-year figure is 5.7% (Palva, Jokinen and Ojala, 1982). Recurrence rates of under 10% at 10 years from surgery can be considered as proof of good surgery and a sound surgical method. Surgeons who have higher rates should give their surgical techniques careful consideration and study the tympanic histopathology in removed specimens.

A proposal (Smyth, 1980) that all patients undergo a second exploratory operation 1 year after primary surgery because of the risk of residual cholesteatoma is not recommended; instead, the technique should be modified so that residual disease becomes rare. As time, costs, hospital facilities, etc. have to be considered, the chosen surgical approach should lie within the capabilities of the average otolaryngologist. Futhermore, performing a second operation does not guarantee that a third operation will not become necessary 1 or 2 years later because of residual disease. I have seen cases where a cholesteatoma pearl 1 mm in diameter is found on the lateral surface of the tympanic membrane in the junctional area 3 years after primary surgery, although there was no indication of cholesteatoma at the 2-year check-up. In all likelihood this could also occur on the medial side of the tympanic membrane.

Long-term follow up results (Ojala, 1979) indicate that hearing deteriorates in ears in which no tympanic reconstruction is made, whereas in reconstructed ears hearing is better after operation than before (although the difference between averages may not be statistically significant). In about 25 to 35% of patients adhesions develop in the middle ear over the years. In these cases the ear can be aerated only by inserting an external ventilation tube. Unfortunately this is not worthwhile in patients who have normal hearing in the other ear (85% of our patients). Results as to social hearing level (30 dB ISO) are shown in *Table 2.1* in 629 ears. It is obvious that the extent of tympanic cleft involvement has a definite effect upon the results and that hearing deteriorates with time.

Table 2.1 Social hearing (30 dB or better, ISO)

	Number of patients	Before surgery	After surgery 1 year	9 years
Mucosa preserved	232	33.2%	56.9%	40.5%
Mucosa removed	397	11.1%	29.0%	20.9%

This discussion concerns only ears in need of extensive surgery and not those requiring only myringoplasty or tympanoplasty. Surgery on ears with severe pathological changes demands experience, perseverance, time and extreme care. It can often take 3 hours to complete an operation and in exceptional cases I may need 4 hours to achieve a satisfactory result. It is therefore difficult to imagine that any surgeon could do more than two operations for chronic ear disease in a day if he is to meet the above requirements, and I think there is cause for concern if a surgeon claims to manage operations on three or four chronically infected ears a day.

References

Beales, P. H. (1959) The problem of the mastoid segment after tympanoplasty. *Journal of Laryngology and Otology*, **73**, 527–531

Guilford, F. R. (1961) Obliteration of the cavity and reconstruction of the auditory canal in temporal bone surgery. *Transactions of the American Academy of Ophthalmology and Otolaryngology*, **65**, 114–122

Jansen, C. (1963) Cartilage-tympanoplasty. *Laryngoscope*, **73**, 1288–1302

Myers, D. and Schlosser, W. D. (1960) Anterior-posterior technique for the treatment of chronic otitis media and mastoiditis. *Laryngoscope*, **70**, 78–83

Ojala, K. (1979) Late results of obliteration in chronic otitis media. MD Thesis, University of Oulu, Finland. *Acta Universitatis Ouluensis*, ser D Medica, **47**

Palva, A., Jokinen, K. and Ojala, K. (1982) Cholesteatoma after radical mastoidectomy with obliteration. *Acta Otolaryngologica (Stockholm)* (in press)

Palva, T. (1963) Surgery of chronic ear without cavity. *Archives of Otolaryngology*, **77**, 570–580

Palva, T. (1973) Operative technique in mastoid obliteration. *Acta Otolaryngologica (Stockholm)*, **75**, 289–290

Palva, T., Karma, P., Kärjä, J. and Palva, A. (1975) Mastoid obliteration. Histopathological study of three temporal bones. *Archives of Otolaryngology*, **101**, 271–275

Palva, T. and Mäkinen, J. (1979) The meatally based musculo-periosteal flap in cavity obliteration. *Archives of Otolaryngology*, **105**, 377–380

Palva, T., Palva, A. and Kärjä, J. (1969) Myringoplasty. *Annals of Otology, Rhinology and Laryngology*, **78**, 1074–1080

Palva, T. and Pulkkinen, K. (1960) Hearing after surgery in chronically discharging ears. II. Radical operation. *Acta Otolaryngologica (Stockholm)*, **52**, 175–185

Smyth, G. D. L. (1980) *Chronic Ear Disease*. New York: Churchill Livingstone

3
Tympanoplasty

Jack Van Doren Hough

For this lecture, I have been asked to discuss some of my personal experiences in dealing with the problems encountered during tympanoplasty and to outline some of the conclusions I have reached in the search for better techniques. I will restrict this discussion to problems referable only to the tympanic membrane and the ossicular chain, and give special emphasis to a technique I have studied carefully and observed over a long period of time.

In the past, like most, I have tried and laid aside many different techniques. This indicates just one thing – dissatisfaction with our results in tympanoplasty. Fortunately, we now find that the common problems and their solutions are related to some very simple principles. Most early techniques, and many still being used today, involve placement of the tympanic membrane graft external to the tympanic membrane remnant. This requires removal of an inordinate amount of squamous epithelium from the tympanic membrane and canal wall. Despite the fact that the bed is created on the external surface, there is insufficient provision for securing the graft to the ossicles and sulcus, thus allowing frequent lateralization of the new tympanic membrane. In addition, many techniques involve the use of artificial materials in the reconstruction of the ossicular chain.

The cardinal principles of the recommended technique are: (1) the use of temporalis fascia medial to the tympanic membrane remnant, medial to the handle of the malleus and medial to the tympanomeatal flap; (2) the preservation of all squamous epithelium of the external ear canal and the tympanic membrane remnant; (3) the use of human ossicles or human bone for reconstruction of the ossicular chain.

I have used this technique consistently for over 17 years in a large number and variety of ears. After this time, I can now strongly recommend this as the standard technique for tympanoplasty. Indeed, its wide acceptance has made it the most commonly performed tympanoplastic procedure today (Hough, 1970).

PROBLEMS AND SOLUTIONS

In the early years, I used onlay grafts of split thickness or full thickness postauricular skin. The use of these materials had to be abandoned rapidly,

30

however, because of the high incidence of dermatitis, reperforation and recurrent cholesteatoma. I then used canal wall skin. Although this was better, all of the difficulties of onlay techniques, regardless of grafting materials, continued to be a plague. Some of the problems I found in using the onlay techniques are described below.

Poor exposure of vital areas of the tympanic cavity

If the squamous epithelium is denuded from the canal wall and tympanic membrane remnant, and the graft simply laid on its external surface, a host of pathological problems within the tympanic cavity may not be recognized. Cholesteatoma, tympanosclerosis, binding adhesions, ossicular necrosis and oto-sclerosis are some of the concomitant problems that may be missed unless the tympanic membrane is elevated and the recesses of the tympanic cavity are thoroughly examined. However, if the underlay technique is used and a wide tympanomeatal flap is elevated with the drum remnant, the entire tympanic cavity is exposed, giving a direct view through the canal.

Blunting of the anterior angle of the tympanic membrane sulcus

This is one of the most unfortunate complications in tympanoplastic healing. If the graft is placed lateral to the tympanic membrane remnant (the onlay technique), it is essential to remove every cell of squamous epithelium from its bed. Otherwise postoperative cholesteatoma will occur. This removal causes the acute angle of the anterior sulcus to have raw surfaces on both areas of the angle. As the graft heals, it is only natural for subcutaneous tissue to build up and obliterate the sharp angle of the anterior sulcus. The tympanic membrane frequently migrates laterally out of the anterior sulcus on to the canal wall. Though this may seem a minor complication, it is often a major cause of hearing loss. The entire region anterior to the handle of the malleus may be splinted, causing great loss of acoustic efficiency. When this occurs, secondary surgical repair becomes extremely difficult even in skilled hands.

The remedy for the blunting or rounding-off of the anterior tympanic membrane is simple. If the graft is placed medial to the tympanic membrane remnant and the squamous epithelium of the anterior sulcus is left intact, a normal angle between the anterior canal wall and the tympanic membrane will be preserved.

Tympanic membrane pull-away from the handle of the malleus

This is another very serious, but preventable, complication in tympanoplasty. The normal self-cleansing migratory pattern of the squamous epithelium in the external ear canal causes it to move gradually toward the exterior. If a tympanic membrane graft is simply placed laterally on the malleus and tympanic membrane remnant, it frequently pulls away from the handle of the malleus toward the isthmus of the canal. The loss of effective vibratory contact, especially at the tip of the handle of the malleus, causes a marked loss of hearing.

The prevention of this problem and its solution is simple – that is, place the graft medial to the handle of the malleus. In this position, it cannot migrate laterally.

Postoperative cholesteatoma from trapped epithelial seed cells

If the graft is to be placed laterally (onlay technique), its new bed must be totally free from squamous epithelial cells. This requires meticulous removal of skin from all areas. This is very difficult, especially in the region of the anterior sulcus, where complete visualization is often impossible. If viable squamous epithelial cells are buried by the onlay graft, insidious development of a hidden cholesteatoma is inevitable.

Again, the solution to this problem is simple – that is, place the graft medial to the squamous epithelium of the tympanic membrane and handle of the malleus. This completely exteriorizes the epithelium so that it is impossible for it to cause postoperative cholesteatoma.

Requirement for excessive epithelial healing

The skin of the external ear canal heals slowly compared to the mucous membrane of the tympanic cavity. Because of this slow squamous epithelial regrowth and the tendency for scar formation as well as graft migration, it is reasonable to save as much squamous epithelium as possible. The onlay technique requires that a large area of normal skin be denuded to provide a good bed for the graft. This needlessly increases the length of time required for the healing of the external layer of the new tympanic membrane. Again, the solution is simple – that is, place the graft under the tympanomeatal flap, under the handle of the malleus and under the entire tympanic membrane remnant. As much healthy squamous epithelium as possible, even on the drum remnant, is preserved. This, therefore, reduces the time needed and the dangers involved in the healing process.

Suitability and availability of the tympanic membrane graft

In the 1950s and early 1960s, the poor results obtained with skin as a tympanic membrane graft were obviously casting a dark cloud on the future of tympanoplasty. Although other connective tissue materials were suggested (vein, perichondrium, homograft dura and cornea, etc.), it was fascia from the external surface of the temporalis muscle that proved to be the most useful.

In selecting a graft, thought must be given to the location of the donor site. Because of the risk of contamination, this should not be in another area of the body. Likewise, there should be a close histological and segmental kinship. The consistency of the graft material is important as well as the amount of tissue available. Other factors, such as ease of surgical removal and comfort for the patient, should also be considered.

In 1961, Storrs published a paper advocating the use of fascia. Almost simultaneously, Ortegren (1964) and Heermann (1962) reported their experience with fascia as a grafting material for the ear, but it was Storrs who was the first to popularize the concept of its use in tympanoplasty.

Today, temporalis fascia is by far the most commonly used tissue for the grafting of the tympanic membrane. It has provided the strong cornerstone necessary for the building of successful results. Temporalis fascia has met our tympanoplastic needs admirably. It is easy to obtain. It occurs within the operative field and it exists in sufficient quantity. It has a low metabolic rate, requiring less nutrition, while being of good consistency. It is histologically adaptable and withstands postoperative infection very well. It even withstands all of the rude things that some of my good colleagues do, such as dry it, cook it, stretch it, mash it, and who knows what else! Most of all, it has by far the finest universal record of permanent perforation closure of any material known. It is from this base that I have combined into a single technique a large number of ideas coming from various sources with some of my own thoughts. When this graft is placed under the tympanomeatal flap under the handle of the malleus and under the tympanic membrane remnant, all of the problems we have previously discussed are solved. I first described this simple technique several years ago (Hough, 1970).

Choice of procedure and preparation

Comprehensive discussion of these items in detail is impossible, but the proper diagnosis, choice of procedure, preoperative preparation, and the care of the patient are obviously basic and extremely important.

A good deal of effort should be made to clear the ear of infection and active inflammation prior to surgery. It may be impossible to stop all discharge completely; nevertheless, a good postoperative course with rapid healing is directly related to the severity of the preoperative active infection. Consideration of the history, audiometric evaluation and careful microscopic assessment of the ear, combined with radiological findings, usually allow one to plan a surgical procedure without later experiencing too many surprises.

The patency and function of the Eustachian tube should be considered, but its postoperative function is impossible to predict by any known test. Careful attention to nasopharyngeal disease and the removal of pathology in the tympanic cavity frequently provide better than expected physiological air exchange to the tympanic cavity via the Eustachian tube. For this reason, an optimistic attitude is justified with regard to Eustachian tube function postoperatively.

The question of whether or not to perform a mastoidectomy at the same time as the tympanoplasty and, if so, whether the canal wall should be left up or taken down is of major importance. Many observations and symptoms are important in this decision. I will emphasize two factors I consider important. Obviously, disease of the mastoid complex has its roots in the tympanic cavity; therefore a careful microscopic study of the upper tympanic cavity and epitympanum is essential. This, combined with the history and the hearing tests, usually provides direct information about the state of the mastoid complex and the ossicular chain. Radiological examination, particularly the conventional Law view of the temporal bone, will provide valuable information not only regarding the surgical anatomy but also regarding the extent of mastoid pneumatization and thus the likely size of the postoperative mastoid bowl should it become necessary to take down the posterior canal wall during tympanomastoidectomy.

Proper preoperative documentation of the patient's history, physical examination and audiometric tests is essential so that future statistical data can be easily processed for review and research, either through keysort cards or a computer system. Only by this careful preservation of recorded information is it possible to assess which procedures are producing the best results in the surgeon's hands. At the same time, it allows comparison of one's own results with those of others and of the efficacy of various procedures and the operator's own skill, thereby providing a basis for further scientific contributions.

TECHNIQUE

At the time of surgery, the scalp is shaved both superiorly and posteriorly to the auricle, and the skin of the scalp is sterilized with a synthetic iodine preparation. If there is a perforation of the tympanic membrane, the solution is not allowed to enter the middle ear. After sufficient sterilization, the ear is cleansed and the area draped.

A generous surgical armamentarium should be provided and its care carefully supervised. A duplicate set of instruments should always be sterile and on hand.

Microscopic study has clearly demonstrated the extreme importance of providing a lint-free physiological environment for the ear, the instruments, the microscope and the materials for grafting. It is incredible how much lint, powder, dust and, probably, bacterial contamination occurs during most surgical procedures. Plastic drapes (to prevent the accumulation of lint), plastic microscope covers, the arrangement of instruments on a plastic-covered instrument table, the use of physiological solutions, etc. are all important.

I will mention a few surgical instruments that I find helpful. I designed a drumscraper for the preparation of the medial side of the tympanic membrane remnant which has proved very useful. Foman upper lateral cartilage scissors (designed for rhinoplasty) can be used to remove temporalis fascia and a Derlacki mobilizer to tuck the graft under the tympanic membrane remnant. Special emphasis is placed on proper suction control throughout the surgical procedure. The Hough-Cadogan (Hough, 1966) foot pedal suction control allows controlled suction (vacuum) so that the suction tip can be used not only to clear blood and secretions, but also to manoeuvre tissues, Gelfoam, etc. into position.

Anesthetic

If an endaural or postauricular mastoidectomy is contemplated, a general anesthetic is used combined with local infiltration. Tympanoplasty alone, i.e. without mastoidectomy, is carried out under local anesthesia, except in children and extremely apprehensive adults. I also use a general anesthetic combined with local anesthesia when there is a marked bony overhang of the anterior canal wall obscuring the tympanic membrane, which will need bone removal. The local anesthetic used is lidocaine 2% (lignocaine; Xylocaine). Approximately 4 ml is injected together with epinephrine 1:100 000 for the scalp and postauricular area, and about 0.75 ml with epinephrine 1:20 000 for the canal interior. This is usually sufficient to provide anesthesia with excellent hemostasis.

Exposure

I prefer a transcanal approach for this operation and do not use a postauricular incision when only a tympanoplasty is to be done. Although good exposure is possible through this incision (and I do not condemn this approach), its disadvantages are obvious. Firstly, the increased burden of healing of the postauricular incision, the soft tissue of the concha, the periosteum and the entire posterior canal wall seems unnecessary. In addition, this procedure prolongs the time necessary for the operation. After waiting for anesthetic infiltration and vasoconstriction, the ear canal and tympanic membrane are exposed to view through the operating microscope. In over 90% of ears, the anterior annulus and/or the rim of the anterior perforation of the tympanic membrane can be seen by tilting the head of the patient or rotating the table and/or adjusting the microscope for a forward view. If this cannot be accomplished, a rectangular section of the skin of the anterior canal wall is removed to be later replaced as a free graft. To do this, an incision is made in the external canal from medial to lateral, beginning approximately 7 mm from the tympanic membrane. Considering the superior point of the tympanic membrane as the twelve o'clock position, in the right ear this incision should be made at about five o'clock. It should be extended laterally to the full length of the ear canal, a little beyond the external portion of the bony canal wall. A second, similar incision should be made parallel, but superiorly, at the one o'clock position. The medial ends of these two parallel incisions should then be joined with the stapes knife. This incision is made approximately 7 mm external and parallel to the anterior tympanic membrane margin. In the same fashion, the lateral ends of the two parallel incisions are joined in the external margin of the canal. Using the sharp stapes knife, the anterior canal wall skin with its periosteum is elevated, beginning medially and rolling the skin and periosteum of the anterior canal wall externally toward the tragus. This skin graft is then placed in a tissue bath, a careful note having been made of its lateral and medial ends as well as its external and internal surfaces so that it may be replaced precisely without changing the skin polarity.

The tissue bath consists simply of a Petri dish containing three pledgets of cotton wool soaked in Physiosol (Abbott Lab.). The tissue can then be placed in the center of the dry Petri dish and the lid replaced. This will keep the tissue moist and physiologically stable until it is ready for use. The tissue should not float in the fluid.

By removing the skin of the anterior canal wall alone, one may gain sufficient exposure of the anterior tympanic membrane remnant to proceed with the tympanoplasty. It may, however, be necessary to remove bone for proper visualization of the drum remnant. While it is not necessary to see the depths of the anterior sulcus since the skin will not be removed in this vital location, a good view of the entire margin of the perforation is essential.

If it is necessary to remove bone, I prefer to use a cutting burr with dry drilling, keeping the burr moving so as not to heat the bone needlessly. To prevent bone dust or chips from entering the middle ear, gelatin sponge (Gelfoam) soaked with Physiosol may be used to completely fill the middle ear medial to the perforation. Suction irrigation may be used, but has the disadvantage that fluid from the external ear canal with bone chips may be washed into the middle ear and mastoid. The potential chemical irritation, contamination, and possible retention of debris caused by the irrigation in my opinion outweighs its advantage.

Preparation of tympanic membrane and graft site

Preparation of the tympanic membrane remnant with preservation of all existing squamous epithelium and of the vital anterior angle is the goal. With the specially designed drumscraper, the underside of the tympanic membrane remnant is scraped thoroughly and the edges of the tympanic membrane remnant at the perforation are rolled out or everted so that areas of squamous ingrowth can be identified. Usually, there is a deep bony niche medial to the sulcus anteriorly and inferiorly. The mucous membrane in this area is denuded in preparation for graft reception. The rolled edges of the perforation contain avascular, scarred, sub-epithelial tissue and should be removed. This is accomplished by inserting a sharp pick through the tympanic membrane remnant approximately 1 mm from the everted perforation margin. The pick is then moved around the edge of the perforation for a few millimeters and repeated incisions of this type are made all around the perforation. The collar thus formed is then removed with cup forceps, assuring a freshened edge of squamous epithelium circumferentially around the margins of the slightly enlarged perforation. The undersurface of the handle of the malleus is scraped and all squamous epithelium removed from this area. However, one need not fear trapping epithelium in this area, since it will be exteriorized by the medial placement of the graft.

Tympanosclerotic plaques of the tympanic membrane are usually removed. These plaques are frequently found in the upper tympanic membrane quadrants. The anterior superior plaques are most apt to cause restriction of the handle of the malleus. Others are usually inconsequential. If a plaque reaches the circumferential edge of the tympanic membrane or attaches to the handle of the malleus, or if it is thick and well formed, it should be removed. One should realize that tympanoscler-osis is a connective-tissue disease not an epithelial disease. It involves only the middle layer of the tympanic membrane and, therefore, these plaques can often be dissected free from the medial side of the squamous epithelium of the tympanic membrane without totally destroying the viable epithelial surface. This is most easily done by using a stapedial 'whirlybird' dissector to elevate the squamous epithelium from the lateral surface of the plaque. Occasionally the plaque must be fractured inward and removed piecemeal. The delicate squamous epithelium on the lateral surface is extremely thin and may be torn. In many instances, however, the fragments of the squamous epithelial sheet may be replaced over the graft once it has been positioned at the end of the operation. This markedly reduces the time of healing required.

Exposure of the tympanic cavity and epitympanum

This is done through a modified stapedectomy incision, using a stapes knife. The incision varies from the routine stapedectomy incision inasmuch as it is placed more laterally or externally as it begins in the superior posterior bony canal wall and is curved toward its inferior arm. This provides a longer, larger flap superiorly for the purpose of better blood supply and also allows sufficient room for bone to be removed from the canal wall in order to expose the necessary portion of the ossicular chain and entry into the epitympanum. This should be done to the extent necessary to fulfil the requirements of ossicular chain repair, removal of tympanosclerosis, and removal of binding or obstructing scar tissue. Furthermore, full exposure of the entry into the epitympanum is necessary to satisfy oneself that there will be physiological aeration of the mastoid complex. By observing the incudostapedial area and its environs, one can determine the health of the mucous membrane of the epitympanum and mastoid complex. The presence or absence of cholesteatoma, cholesterol granulosis, etc. can easily be determined.

It is my belief that oftentimes the surgeon's uncertainty concerning the epitympanum and mastoid complex results in unnecessary mastoidectomies. With adequate exposure (*see above*), one can detect with certainty the presence or absence of significant disease, because one has a clear view of the base area from which it arises. I object to the procedure of posterior tympanotomy in which essentially normal mastoid cells are removed and the tympanic cavity is visualized horizontally through a small facial recess opening. This is a needless, time-consuming and dangerous procedure, particularly when a good transcanal exposure of the vital incudostapedial area can be so easily and quickly obtained.

Removal of pathological sequelae from the tympanum

After proper exposure, various constricting scar bands and tympanosclerotic plaques are removed from the tympanic membrane and cavity. The most frequent scar band of importance stretches from the promontory to the tip of the handle of the malleus. This scar band should be cut short at both ends and removed. The handle of the malleus should not be shortened. To prevent re-scarring, it is usually necessary to place a small piece of Gelfilm (Upjohn) between these two raw surfaces as one of the last steps of the operation.

The management of tympanosclerotic plaques around the ossicles requires skill and judgement. These plaques should be removed, if possible, so that all ossicles are freely moveable. Those areas that cannot safely be released should be bypassed by ossicular grafting. Care must be used in the removal of plaques around the stapes. A break in the footplate or the annular ligament is considered to be a serious complication. For this reason, removal of scar tissue and tympanosclerosis in this area should be the last step in the operation. If in doubt, the operation should be staged.

Obtaining the fascial graft to reconstruct the tympanic membrane

To obtain the fascial graft, I make an incision in the scalp in an anterior–posterior direction approximately 3 cm long and 3 cm above the superior attachment of the external auricle. The dissection is carried down to the superficial layer of the temporalis fascia. All loose areolar tissue is elevated in a wide area over the external surface of the fascia for a distance of about 5 cm. A small incision is then made in the fascia near the level of the original incision, and, with an elevator, the fascia is then elevated on its medial surface from the temporalis muscle over approximately the same area. I have found that curved Foman upper lateral cartilage rhinoplasty scissors are excellent for removal of the fascia. A large piece of fascia is obtained and placed in the moist tissue chamber. The graft should not be allowed to dry. It should not be pressed or handled with the fingers. Procedures that deliberately alter the chemistry of the graft should not be used. To dry the graft out like parchment is certainly not physiological.

When the graft is ready for use, it is removed from the moist tissue chamber and placed on a green Teflon block where all excess tissue is removed. It is then cut to the proper size and shape. If the perforation is in the anterior tympanic membrane or if the total tympanic membrane is to be reconstructed, the graft size should be approximately 25×18 mm. If only the posterior portion of the tympanic membrane is to be reconstructed, the graft need only be 20×18 mm in size.

A piece of compressed Gelfoam slightly smaller than the size of the tympanic membrane is then cut and placed on the graft in the area corresponding to the planned new tympanic membrane. If there is to be ossicular grafting, a pie-shaped piece of Gelfoam is cut away in this area before placement of the graft. A small cut in the graft along the place where the handle of the malleus will be resting may need to be made in order to provide a triangular flap so that it can be folded back to expose the posterior superior quadrant of the tympanic cavity for ossicular grafting at the end of the surgical procedure. After repairing the ossicular chain, this fascial flap can be replaced to seal the posterior superior tympanic membrane finally.

The graft with its Gelfoam backing is then inserted into the tympanic cavity so that the Gelfoam provides an internal bed in the middle ear for the new tympanic membrane. Its dry compressed stiffness also allows maneuvering of the graft. The anterior edge is placed first under the handle of the malleus; the graft with the Gelfoam backing is then pushed forward until the posterior edge of the Gelfoam sponge is well in the middle ear. The trailing edge of the graft is spread out over the exposed bone of the posterior superior bony canal wall so that it covers the bone to the line of the original tympanotomy incision. The tympanomeatal flap is then replaced over the graft, thus securing the posterior half of the graft.

The last area that needs attention is anteriorly under the anterior sulcus. The tympanic cavity is deeper in the Eustachian tube region, and frequently it is necessary to provide better medial support for the graft in this area in order to keep it from falling into the middle ear. Working through the perforation, the anterior edge of the graft is lifted out from under the anterior tympanic membrane remnant and folded on itself by rolling it laterally and posteriorly to expose the underlying gelatin sponge. Pledgets of absorbable Gelfoam soaked with Physiosol may then be properly positioned in all directions. These additional pieces will build up a proper bed for the fascia so that it is in good apposition to the medial surface of the drum remnant. Following this, the graft is replaced as far under the superior, anterior and inferior annulus of the tympanic membrane remnant as possible. The tympanic membrane remnant and the thin external epithelial sheet of cells near its edge can then be teased back into position over the graft so as to reduce the time of healing. The ear canal is then filled with Gelfoam pledgets soaked with Physiosol. I have not found that antibiotic or anti-inflammatory steroid solutions are necessary.

Special mention should be made of those cases in which there is a total absence of the tympanic membrane or even the fibrous annulus. It is my experience that the above procedure is highly successful even in these ears. There is always an opportunity to denude mucous membrane under the bony ledge of the anterior and inferior annulus. Even the lateral margin of the Eustachian tube orifice may be denuded. If the graft is properly placed in this anterior niche area, the squamous epithelial cells along the anterior margin of the canal wall will quickly bind the graft in position. Re-perforation is extremely rare. I am convinced that if re-perforation does occur, it is usually due to improper placement of the graft.

Placement of ossicular grafts and Gelfilm

In those cases in which the ossicular chain must be reconstructed, the tympanomeatal flap with the graft is again elevated to expose the posterior superior tympanic cavity. A small cut in the upper edge of the fascial graft adjacent to the long process of the malleus (*see above*) will have already been made prior to graft insertion. This cut should extend about two-thirds of the distance toward the tip of the handle of the malleus. This linear incision allows one to fold the fascial graft back like a tent flap, exposing the posterior superior tympanic cavity. The ossicles are then placed in good position and held in place by a Gelfoam cast. If desired, Gelfilm discs or strips may be appropriately placed to prevent scar bands.

Results

An intact, mobile, and normally shaped tympanic membrane can be obtained in an extremely high proportion of ears treated with this technique. Most well-trained otologists report long-term success in 95 to 99% of cases. In my last reported series of 773 ears, 98.9% had long-term perforation closure. I believe that if one is not obtaining a rate of over 90% closure the technique is faulty (Hough, 1958, 1963, 1977)

OSSICULAR RECONSTRUCTION

In those cases in which there is discontinuity of the ossicular chain, the surgeon may choose from a variety of materials to bridge the gap. Today those possibilities include plastics, metals, ceramics, cartilage and human bone. Although I have tried most of those suggested, since 1956 I have used primarily human ossicles or bone in rebuilding the ossicular chain. It was at that time that I encountered a case of complete incudostapedial joint separation. Since no reconstructive techniques had yet been devised, I used a small bone graft taken from the edge of the canal wall to fill the space between the two bones. This first tympanic cavity bone graft did survive and the result was excellent. Because of this, I, along with many other otologists, have searched continuously for better methods of utilizing human material for ossicular reconstruction.

During the ensuing years, a host of other new ideas arose among otologists for solving problems of ossicular chain separation. Most innovators suggested using plastic or metal prostheses. The rapidity of the appearance of new designs and materials during the past 20 years has been startling. This continued change, both in prostheses and in techniques of application, is to me strong evidence of continued dissatisfaction with short- and long-term results. Unfortunately, almost all of the prostheses used during the 1960s, with the exception of prostheses used in stapedectomy, caused erosion, became displaced, or were extruded within a matter of weeks, months or years. I have tried most of these prostheses and have seen unfortunate results both in my own patients and in those of many of my colleagues. Because of this experience, I, as well as others, have continued to try to improve the rate of success in bone grafts.

In the late 1950s, Hall and Rytzner (1957) suggested a number of autograft arrangements whereby the conductive bridge could be rebuilt. During this time I found that the long process and body of the incus, with the short process cut off, could be used to connect the malleus with the footplate of the stapes. A major step forward was the interposition of the body of the incus on the head of the stapes to connect it with the malleus and the tympanic membrane (House, Patterson and Linthicum, 1966). This interposition technique, combined with my successful experience in using the long process of the incus from the footplate of the stapes to the malleus, provided a working basis for the reconstruction of almost all ossicular chain defects with human bone as grafts. In the mid-1960s, many of us also began using homograft bone for reconstruction. There seemed to be no difference in biocompatibility between homograft and autograft bone. This discovery provided the possibility for each surgeon to have a bone bank to meet all needs. During this time, only minor trimming or alterations of the bone grafts was done, and as a result many grafts shifted out of position, causing poor hearing. This acted as a stimulus for modification of the size and shape of the ossicular graft. In 1972, Pennington (1977) presented the first major idea for sculpturing grafts for better joint coupling and stability. Many of us have continued to further model these grafts so as to reduce the bulk and provide better permanent linkage.

Also, refinements in porous plastics in the early 1970s have produced a new generation of ossicular replacement prostheses (Shea, 1977). Ceramics have also been added to the range of options. Because of the poor results with prostheses in the past, these new artificial materials must be shown to provide better long-term results than our present good results with human bone grafts before we adopt them for general use.

Classification of ossicular chain defects and their correction

To ensure an orderly approach to the various conductive problems in the ear and their correction, I use the following classification (Hough, 1977).

Incudostapedial joint separation, with long process of incus usually missing (*type I*)

This requires reconstruction from the head of the stapes to the handle of the malleus. The incus is by far the most vulnerable portion of the ossicular chain and it remains the commonest cause of interruption of the ossicular chain for many well-recognized reasons.

TECHNIQUE
I believe this problem is best corrected by using either an autograft or homograft sculptured ossicle to be inserted between the head of the stapes and the handle of the malleus (*Figure 3.1*). The technique of sculpturing I find most helpful is to first

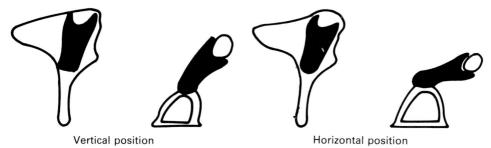

Vertical position   Horizontal position

Figure 3.1 Reconstruction from the head of the stapes to the malleus, using a sculptured incus (autograft or homograft)

carefully measure the distance between the handle of the malleus and the head of the stapes. If the distance is very short, the patient's own head of the malleus may be used. In this instance, the neck of the malleus may be cut with a House-Dieter malleus nipper, and the head and neck removed from the epitympanum. The bone is grasped with good bone-holding forceps (Sheehy or Derlacki). Using a large diamond burr, the neck is flattened. A pocket for the reception of the head of the stapes is then drilled with a small burr. At the opposite end of the bone (the superior edge of the head of the malleus), a saddle indentation is made to clamp around the handle of the host malleus. The bone is then reduced in size with a large diamond burr until these two effective joint ends are connected with a cylindrical shaft of bone (Hough, 1977).

Most frequently, however, the distance to be spanned between the head of the stapes and the handle of the malleus is too long to use the head of the malleus. In this case the body of the incus may be used (either autograft or homograft). The short process is grasped with bone forceps, and the long process is cut off with a large diamond burr, producing a flat surface against the inferior side of the body of the incus. With a smaller burr, a deep indentation is made, slightly larger than the head of the stapes. On the opposite end (the superior edge of the body of the incus), a saddle indentation is made for the reception of the handle of the malleus. The bone is then reduced in size and sculptured for a precise firm fit (Hough, 1977). The sculptured bone graft is then placed in the ear so that connection is made with the malleus first. With a right angle pick or hoe inserted into the niche made for the stapes, the graft couple with the malleus is pushed forward until the stapes head can be encased by the indentation on the end of the graft. The spring tension produced by holding the malleus forward is then released, providing a very secure bridge between the two bones. A cast of wet Gelfoam pledgets can then be placed around the graft, but this is usually not necessary.

RESULTS

In a recent study of a large series of ears with this type of defect, I have compared the results of combined ossicular chain reconstruction and reconstruction of the tympanic membrane with a fascial graft to those in which no tympanic membrane grafting was carried out. Correction of the ossicular defect alone, using the technique described above, resulted in long-term hearing improvement to within 10 dB of the preoperative bone conduction in the three speech frequencies in 86.5% of cases; in 89.5% hearing was restored to social adequacy (Hough, 1977). In those ears in which the tympanic membrane was grafted during the same operation in which the ossicular chain was reconstructed in the above fashion, only 7% less closed the air–bone gap to within 10 dB of the preoperative bone conduction in the three speech frequencies (Hough, 1977). Therefore, even the simultaneous grafting of the tympanic membrane and the ossicular chain obtains a high degree of success. Furthermore, even if the ossicular graft fails, the stage is set for a secondary procedure, since one will then be working in an essentially normal tympanic cavity with an intact tympanic membrane. I therefore feel that this is a strong encouragement not to deliberately stage these procedures.

Absence of the arch of the stapes (*type II*)

This requires reconstruction from the footplate of the stapes to the handle of the malleus. In my experience, absence of the arch of the stapes is almost always accompanied by the loss of the long process of the incus. In this event, an autograft is not possible. The short process plus the body of the incus is not large enough to bridge the span between the handle of the malleus and the stapedial footplate. For this reason, I choose a homograft incus or handle of a malleus, preferably the latter (*Figure 3.2*).

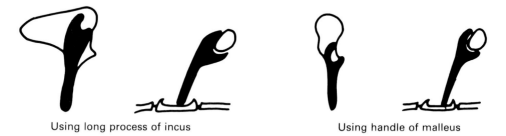

Using long process of incus   Using handle of malleus

Figure 3.2 Reconstruction from the footplate of the stapes to the malleus, using a long process of incus (*left*) or the handle of a malleus (*right*)

In 1958 I encountered an ear in which the superstructure of the stapes had been destroyed by lightning. The problem was to reconstruct the sound-conducting bridge from the oval window to the handle of the malleus. As prostheses were unknown at that time, I was forced to use the materials at hand. The long process of the incus was still in good condition, therefore the incus was removed from the attic, the short process was cut off with Lempert malleus nippers and the long process was placed in the oval window. The articulating face of the incus was then rested against the handle of the malleus. This produced an excellent permanent hearing improvement and has provided the basis of our present approach to this problem. We have modified this by using extensive sculpturing introduced by Pennington (1977) and find this to be of great value.

TECHNIQUE
The distance between the handle of the malleus and the footplate of the stapes is carefully measured.

If using the malleus, the head of the homograft malleus is grasped with the bone holder, and with a small diamond burr the normal indentation in the neck of the malleus just superior to the lateral process is deepened to make a saddle-shaped receptacle for the host handle of the malleus. The bone of the head and neck is then drilled away. The saddle-cup of the graft is then placed around the medial surface of the host malleus and forceps are used to place the opposite end, or the tip of the bone graft, in the center of the footplate of the stapes. If the oval window margins on the promontory or facial ridge have been denuded of mucous membrane, it is advisable to place small triangular pieces of Gelfilm between the graft and the oval window margins to prevent fixation. Also, with this graft placement, it is wise to provide a cast of fluid-soaked Gelfoam pledgets completely surrounding the homograft.

When using a homograft incus, the short process of the incus is grasped firmly by bone-holding forceps and the long process is thinned with a large diamond burr. An indentation saddle for the reception of the handle of the malleus is made on the body of the incus. This is usually best placed on the slope of the superior edge of the body of the incus toward the short process. The remainder of the block of bone is then sculptured into a long cylindrical shaft using a large diamond burr. A length is then cut off at the tip of the long process with Lempert malleus nippers to correspond exactly to the measurement desired. The cupped saddle end of the graft is then placed around the medial surface of the handle of the malleus and the shaft rotated to rest in the center of the stapedial footplate. A cast of wet Gelfoam pledgets is then placed around the bone graft to secure it in position until healed (Hough, 1977).

RESULTS

Even though this graft is not tightly secured at the footplate and spans the entire depth of the tympanic cavity, results are very commendable. My recent series showed that if there is no significant tympanic cavity pathology, the air–bone gap is closed to within 10 dB of the preoperative bone conduction in the three speech frequencies in 73.3%; 93% obtained excellent improvement. Significant tympanic cavity pathology (such as cholesteatoma, tympanosclerosis, etc.) requiring extensive surgery, usually combined with mastoidectomy, obviously increases the possibility of failure. Of these cases, 51.9% closed the air–bone gap to within 10 dB, and another 26.4%, although not closing the air–bone gap to within 10 dB, were restored to adequate social hearing (speech reception threshold, SRT below 40 dB), making an excellent improvement in 77.4% of ears with this extensive repair. This evidence clearly contradicts the premise that these patients should have a planned second-stage operation.

Absence of the total stapes, including the footplate (*type III*)

This is usually accompanied by absence of the long process of the incus and requires construction from the open oval window to the handle of the malleus. Obviously this condition does not occur in an ear with a perforation of the tympanic membrane, since labyrinthitis would certainly occur and destroy the inner ear through the open vestibule; therefore, in this case, we are not dealing with an ear requiring a simultaneous tympanic membrane graft, but with ears with an intact tympanic membrane requiring stapedectomy and complete repair of the ossicular chain from the open oval window to the handle of the malleus. If, however, during repair of the tympanic membrane, complete stapedial ankylosis is found, this is the cardinal indication to stage the operation, i.e. to repair the tympanic membrane and plan a second operation with a type III tympanoplasty for a later date.

TECHNIQUE

This condition may be corrected by the method suggested for type II, but with the additional removal of the footplate of the stapes and the sealing of the oval window with a perichondrial graft.

Victor Goodhill (1974) first introduced the use of perichondrium in stapedectomy. Tragal perichondrium is an ideal graft material for the oval window when the footplate has been fractured or expelled from the oval window due to trauma or during stapedectomy. Unlike other graft materials used over the oval window, such as vein or fascia, perichondrium is stiff enough to prevent the ossicular graft from falling into the vestibule. Perichondrium can easily be obtained by making an incision over the tragus and removing the dome of the tragal cartilage. The perichondrium is then removed from the cartilage and trimmed to the correct size to seal the oval window.

A homograft ossicle, either a sculptured handle of the malleus or a sculptured long process of the incus, is then placed in the center of the graft. The opposite end is cupped around the handle of the malleus and Gelfoam cast applied.

RESULTS

In the recent series of patients mentioned above, the long-term results were as follows: 83.3% closed the air–bone gap to within 10 dB of the preoperative bone conduction; in an additional 8.4% hearing was restored to social adequacy (SRT under 40 dB). Fortunately, none of these ears were made worse in this particular series. Although this group is small in number compared to the other types mentioned, it is obvious that in a clean, healthy ear with an intact tympanic membrane extensive ossicular chain reconstruction may be carried out with a high degree of success.

Absence of the incus, malleus and tympanic membrane, with the stapes and its superstructure still intact (*type IV*)

This requires reconstruction of all three structures. The principal problem faced here is the missing handle of the malleus. This occurs much less frequently than loss of the long process of the incus or of the superstructure of the stapes and presents a more difficult problem.

TECHNIQUE

In this type of reconstruction, it is my practice to use a fascial graft to reconstruct the tympanic membrane in precisely the same manner as mentioned above. The underlay technique is used. Once the fascia has been properly placed on a Gelfoam bed and the tympanomeatal flap returned to a good position over it, the tympanic membrane remnant with the tympanomeatal flap and the fascial graft is lifted from posterior to anterior, exposing the posterior half of the tympanic cavity. A shaft of homograft bone (either ossicular or cortical bone) approximately the size of the handle of the malleus is then placed on the medial surface of the fascial graft. A homograft handle of a malleus with a small area of attached homograft tympanic membrane is also ideal for this ossicular graft. Its position should be similar to that of the original host handle of the malleus. Attachment to the medial surface of the fascial graft is not a problem: like an octopus, the fascia immediately adheres to it and holds it in place (Hough, 1977).

The other bone graft is then placed from this newly grafted malleus to the stapedial head, as in type I, and a Gelfoam cast is used to hold everything in position. The graft is then laid on the bone of the posterior superior canal wall and the tympanomeatal flap is returned to its original position over it (Hough, 1977).

RESULTS

Despite the complex reconstruction, the results in our series were very encouraging. The air–bone gap was closed to within 10 dB of the preoperative bone conduction in the three speech frequencies in 66.6% of ears without significant active tympanic cavity pathology (Hough, 1977).

Absence of the stapes superstructure, incus, malleus and tympanic membrane, with only the footplate of the stapes remaining (*type V*)

The tympanic membrane, the handle of the malleus, the incus and the stapedial superstructure all require reconstruction because they are either missing or damaged beyond use. This entails: (1) reconstruction of the tympanic membrane with a fascial graft; (2) reconstruction of the handle of the malleus as above; and (3) reconstruction of the ossicular chain from the stapedial footplate to the grafted handle of the malleus as in type II.

RESULTS

For all of these structures to remain in perfect position throughout healing is a difficult requirement. Nevertheless, of 39 ears in which this reconstruction was carried out in a single procedure (many with concomitant or superimposed tympanic cavity and mastoid pathology), 48.7% closed the air–bone gap to within 10 dB of the preoperative bone conduction in the three speech frequencies and 59% returned socially adequate hearing (Hough, 1977). I will emphasize again that these techniques frequently provide a success in a single procedure. If not, that is if the bony bridge between the new malleus graft and the oval window shifts out of contact in healing, one still has the new handle of the malleus attached to an intact tympanic membrane as a cornerstone ready for a second-stage reconstruction. In other words, one has nothing to lose and everything to gain by trying to complete the total reconstruction in one operation rather than planning a two-stage procedure from the outset.

Finally, may I summarize the reasons for choosing sculptured ossicles instead of prosthetic devices. Firstly, human bone grafted into the tympanic cavity undergoes quick reconstitution; it is covered with protective mucous membrane and becomes part of the body. The bone becomes vascularized and viable, whereas in the case of artificial prostheses the mucous membrane can never become a living part of the prosthetic material. Though newer artificial plastic material may be porous, it remains a foreign body to which the organism has an aversion which may range from mild to intense. Secondly, although the biological incompatibility may be mild in newer plastics, the reaction continues over a period of years and may finally lead to rejection. During this process, necrosis of the bone to which it is attached may cause looseness and gradual loss of hearing. Thirdly, regarding functional results, the burden of proof is on those who advocate the use of prostheses. They must be able to show that improvement in hearing is not only as good, but even better than with ossicular grafts, and that it can be maintained in the long-term, i.e. over at least 5–10 years. Remember, we already know that the long-term functional results with human bone are good. If, indeed, the new generation of porous plastics and ceramics can be shown to exceed all of the specifications I have mentioned, we will join our patients in happy acclaim. Meanwhile, objective, honest, scientific appraisal should be the rule.

SUMMARY

Today's otological surgeon, despite the delicate and complex problems he faces, may approach the reconstruction of the tympanic membrane and ossicular chain with proven techniques. If the basic principle of placing the fascial graft medial to the handle of the malleus, medial to the tympanic membrane remnant and medial to the tympanomeatal flap is observed, the rate of perforation closure will be extremely high. Furthermore, the results of ossicular chain reconstruction are also very good if sculptured human ossicles are used. Although encouraging results have made these techniques acceptable, many pathological problems, such as atelectasis, tympanosclerosis and chronic epithelial diseases, remain and present an unremitting challenge which prevents complacency.

References

Goodhill, V. (1974) Posterior arch stapedioplasty. Ten commandments for stapedectomy. *Archives of Otolaryngology*, **100**, 460–464

Hall, A. and Rytzner, C. (1957) Stapedectomy and autotransplantation of ossicles. *Acta Otolaryngologica*, **47**, 318

Heermann, J. (1962) Erfahrungen mit frei transplantiertem Faszienbindegewebe des musculus temporalis bei Tympanoplastik und Verkleinerung der Radikalhöhle. Knorpelbrücke vom stapes zum unteren Trommelfellrand. *Zeitschrift für Laryngologie, Rhinologie und Otologie (Stuttgart)*

Hough, J. V. D. (1958) Malformations and anatomical variations seen in the middle ear during the operation for mobilization of the stapes. *Laryngoscope*, **68**, 1337–1379

Hough, J. V. D. (1963) Congenital malformations of the middle ear. *Archives of Otolaryngology*, **78**, 335–343

Hough, J. V. D. (1966) Suction control with a footpedal. *Transactions of the American Academy of Ophthalmology and Otolaryngology*, **70**, 846–847

Hough, J. V. D. (1970) Tympanoplasty with the interior fascial graft technique and ossicular reconstruction. *Laryngoscope*, **80,** 1358–1413

Hough, J. V. D. (1976) Panel on tympanic membrane grafting. *Fifth Shambaugh International Workshop*

Hough, J. V. D. (1977) Techniques for incus necrosis and results: ossicular reconstruction. In *Proceedings of the Sixth Shambaugh International Workshop on Otomicrosurgery and Third Shea Fluctuant Hearing Loss Symposium* (Huntsville, Alabama, 1977), edited by G. E. Shambaugh, Jr. and J. J. Shea, pp. 422–429. Huntsville Ala.: Strode Publishers

House, W. F., Patterson, M. E. and Linthicum, F. H. (1966) Incus homografts in chronic ear surgery. *Archives of Otolaryngology*, **84,** 148–153

Ortegren, U. (1964) Myringoplasty. Four years' experience of temporal fascial grafts. *Acta Otolaryngologica*, **193** (Suppl.), 1–43

Pennington, C. L. (1977) Incus interposition techniques. In *Proceedings of the Shambaugh Fifth International Workshop on Middle Ear Microsurgery and Fluctant Hearing Loss* (Huntsville, Alabama, 1977), edited by G. E. Shambaugh, Jr. and J. J. Shea, pp. 323–334. Huntsville Ala. Strode Publishers

Shea, J. (1977) Plastipore and proplast implants in tympanoplasty. In *Proceedings of the Shambaugh Fifth International Workshop on Middle Ear Microsurgery and Fluctant Hearing Loss* (Huntsville, Alabama, 1977), edited by G. E. Shambaugh, Jr. and J. J. Shea, pp. 352–355. Huntsville Ala.: Strode Publishers

Storrs, L. A. (1961) Myringoplasty with the use of fascia grafts. *Archives of Otolaryngology*, **74,** 45–49

4
Middle ear transformer reconstruction
Mansfield F. W. Smith

This course summarizes the author's experience with otologic freeze-dried, ethylene oxide sterilized allografts (homografts) since 1968.

Allograft reconstruction of the middle ear transformer is not difficult and affords a like-for-like replacement of missing parts. Allografts also afford a logical system of middle ear and external osseous canal reconstruction by providing a similar biological and anatomical replacement when autograft material is not available. An otologic allograft sterilized by ethylene oxide and freeze-dried is an attractive alternative to the use of chemically fixed or prosthetic alloplasts. It has the inherently superior mechanical design of an allograft as well as minimal donor tissue physiochemical alteration. Moreover, it is capable of more normal metabolic and mechanical function, and has a more normal histological structure and gross anatomical appearance. In addition, it may be reliably remodeled and repaired (Smith, 1980).

The great variation in surgical techniques of middle ear reconstruction, and the multitude of metal and plastic prostheses available for ossicular replacement, testify to the difficulty of this type of reconstruction and to the lack of uniform results. Extrusion, displacement, loss of continuity and fixation are common recurrent problems following ossicular chain reconstruction.

LITERATURE REVIEW

Since the report of Matte (1901) of a myringostapediopexy, numerous methods have been employed to bridge the gap between the tympanic membrane and the labyrinthine fluids. Initial reconstructive efforts, such as those of Hall and Rytzner (1957), focused on the use of autogenous materials. Jansen (1958) in 1956 and House *et al.* (1966) used homologous cartilage and ossicles respectively in the reconstruction of the ossicular chain.

Despite many excellent short- and long-term results (Guilford, 1965; Smyth and Kerr, 1967) with autogenous and homologous prostheses, the success of polyethylene and Teflon pistons in stapes surgery focused attention on the potential role of synthetic biocompatible materials in ossicular chain reconstruction. The otologic literature of the early 1960s contains a number of case reports outlining the use of polyethylene prostheses of various shapes and sizes in the restoration of ossicular continuity (DeSebastian, 1960; Glaninger, 1964). Interspersed with these articles are reports of early and late extrusions, especially in cases requiring contact of the prosthesis with the tympanic membrane or graft (Sheehy, 1965; Siedentop and Brown, 1966).

In 1974 Shea introduced a polytetrafluoroethylene-vitreous carbon prosthesis (Proplast) designed to present the tympanic membrane with a 'soft gradual interphase of low modulus to overcome the problems of displacement, extrusion, and absorption' (Shea and Homsy, 1974). Although 1-year follow-up studies revealed an extrusion rate of only 2%, this material was supplanted in 1978 by a high-density polyethylene sponge prosthesis (Plastipore) which, according to Shea and Emmett (1978), 'was superior to the prosthesis made of Proplast'.

Despite encouraging short-term results, problems with extrusion persisted (Strauss, 1979). The placement of cartilage between the prosthesis and the tympanic membrane to prevent extrusion has been described by a number of surgeons using this method. Sheehy (1978) has reported excellent results. However, in a long-term study by Smyth (1982), a 57% failure rate in restoring hearing was noted with the use of partial ossicular replacement prostheses (PORPs) and a 78% failure rate with total ossicular replacement prostheses (TORPs). Further, the

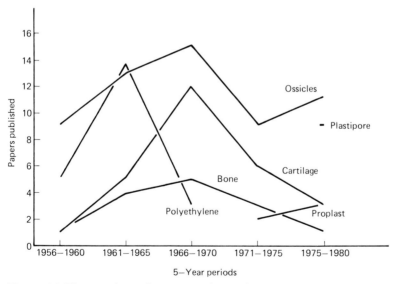

Figure 4.1 The number of papers written about each type of ossicular reconstructive material, in 5-year blocks over 25 years

proportion of unsatisfactory results increased with the passage of time. Smyth reported an 11% extrusion rate. Kerr (1981) has recently reported electron microscopic evidence of giant cell digestion of porous polyethylene when used as an ossicular replacement in the human middle ear.

There is a paucity of long-term reports with any type of ossicular chain reconstruction. It is evident that there have been a number of changes in techniques and materials in ossicular reconstruction, but few reports as to why. *Figure 4.1* gives some indication of the changing trends in ossicular chain reconstruction. The analysis is based on the number of papers written about each type of ossicular reconstructive material in 5-year periods over 25 years. The materials considered are ossicles, bone, cartilage, and three synthetic materials – polyethylene, Proplast and Plastipore.

Freeze-dried otologic orthotopic allografts, because of their superior mechanical design and minimal physiochemical alteration of donor tissue, offer an attractive alternative to the use of alloplasts and chemically fixed or heat-processed ossicular grafts.

The advantages of allograft bone over alloplastic materials (metals/plastics) depend upon host acceptance and viability of the implant. Controversy is evident in the variety of techniques which exist for processing ossicular grafts, including autoclaving, freezing, freeze-drying, and insertion (or soaking) in organic mercurials, formalin and alcohol.

Based on animal and clinical research, freeze-dried bone and fibrous tissue are stable transplants when stored in vacuum, function similarly to an autograft, and retain their original molecular structure. Grafts can be stored at room temperature as long as the vacuum is retained (Smith, 1980).

PROCUREMENT

The process begins with procurement of the otologic allografts. The temporal bone cores are removed from the refrigerated cadaver within 24 hours of death. Only temporal bones free from neoplasm or infection are selected. There are no donor age limits.

The temporal bone cores are removed from the cadaver under clean, but not aseptic, conditions, Cores are surface-decontaminated with an iodorphor solution (povidone-iodine, Betadine) and rinsed repeatedly with sterile 0.9% saline solution until the washings are clear. Cores are stored at 4 °C for no longer than 14 days in isotonic saline.

PROCESSING

Ethylene oxide sterilization and freeze-drying are carried out in the following manner:

(1) The temporal bone is dissected, and the de-epithelialized tympanic membrane and periosteal cuff and attached malleus, incus and stapes are removed together or separately.
(2) Graft tissue is placed in a container in which it is gas-sterilized. The 10% ethylene oxide/90% carbon dioxide gas sterilization is carried out in an

ethylene oxide sterilizer (Steri-Vac, 3M Company, Model 400) at 29.4 °C. The gas sterilization is performed under vacuum, which allows the gas to permeate the tissue thoroughly (duration: 4½ hours).

(3) The graft is prefrozen to −70 °C in a two-stage freezer for at least 1 hour. The graft may be stored indefinitely in this state.

(4) The bottles containing grafts are transferred to the freeze-dryer (VerTis, Model 25 SRC) using aseptic precautions. The grafts are freeze-dried for 5 days with the condenser temperature set at −56 °C and the shelf temperature set at 20 °C. This prolonged freeze-drying ensures a low water content and dramatically reduces the residual levels of ethylene oxide and its hydrolysis products left in the tissue.

(5) The allograft containers are sealed. Test samples that underwent the same processing are cultured. The culture reports are available in 24 hours.

Ethylene oxide is used for sterilization because it is an effective agent against all micro-organisms and causes no identifiable tissue alteration. Sterile, non-toxic tissue implants are produced by this process.

Ethylene oxide is a colorless gas at ordinary room temperatures; it liquefies readily at 10.9 °C and freezes at −111.3 °C. This chemical not only dissolves in ordinary solvents, including water, but also permeates solids from which unreacted ethylene oxide is slowly released. An inherent disadvantage of ethylene oxide is the fact that it or its breakdown products are retained (Rosomoff, 1959). Work at the Bone Transplant Unit of the Northern California Transplant Bank has demonstrated that residual concentration of ethylene oxide and its toxic by-products are satisfactorily reduced following prolonged lyophilization. In addition, the depth of penetration of ethylene oxide necessary for sterilization of otologic transplants further reduces the potential for toxicity.

CLINICAL APPLICATIONS OF FREEZE-DRIED OTOLOGIC ALLOGRAFTS

Tympanic membrane with malleus

Fibrous tympanic membrane with attached long process of the malleus and periosteal cuff is used in two situations: (1) intact posterior osseous canal and (2) open mastoid cavity.

Intact posterior osseous canal

The de-epithelialized fibrous tympanic membrane with attached periosteal cuff is used to position the malleus neck over the oval window. The head of the malleus is removed, but a portion of the neck may remain to decrease the distance between the malleus and the head, or the footplate, of the stapes. Slightly more of the posterior osseous canal is removed than in a stapedectomy procedure to allow rotation of the malleus neck over the oval window.

At a second stage procedure, 6 months following insertion of the tympanic membrane and malleus, a partial ossicular replacement allograft (PORA) is placed between the malleus neck and stapes head or footplate.

The periosteal cuff is incised at the six and twelve o'clock positions to allow more accurate placement of the periosteal cuff against the denuded osseous canal. In most instances the external auditory canal periosteum and epithelial membrane are window-shaded laterally and then placed back over the cuff and fibrous tympanic membrane graft. The ideal covering of the tympanic membrane portion of the graft is epithelium from the auditory canal. The graft and canal flaps are then held in position with Gelfoam pledgets soaked in a 10% chloramphenicol (Chloromycetin) solution (steroids may delay healing and epithelial covering of the graft).

The open mastoid cavity

The tympanic membrane graft with periosteal cuff and attached long process of the malleus may be used to convert the radical mastoid middle ear to a modified radical mastoid. The malleus head is removed and the neck rotated close to the head of the stapes if present and, if not, to approximately the same position. Incisions are made in the periosteal membrane at the six and twelve o'clock positions, and the periosteal membrane is trimmed so that approximately 4 mm extends up the denuded anterior osseous canal.

Partial ossicular replacement allograft (PORA)

The ossicular replacement allografts are used to span defects between the neck of the malleus and the head or mobile footplate of the stapes. Reliable reconstruction of the middle ear transformer requires that the neck of the malleus be positioned over the oval window. Ossicular replacement allografts come in various sizes and are measured from the end or central portion of the acetabulum to the center of the crutch. It is expected that these replacement allografts may need some modification

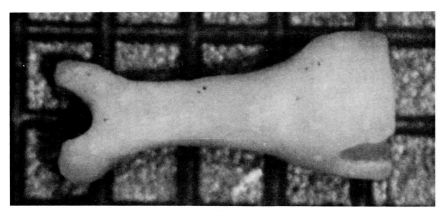

Figure 4.2 Crutch and acetabulum: configuration 2–3.5 mm

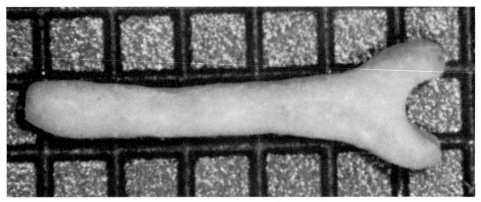

Figure 4.3 Partial ossicular replacement allograft: configuration 3.5–5 mm

by the surgeon to adjust to the specific requirements of each patient. These allografts are homotropic in that they are fashioned from human ossicles. They are supplied in sizes from 2 to 5 mm; from 2 to 3 mm in 0.25 mm increments and from 3 to 5 mm in 0.5 mm increments (*Figures 4.2 and 4.3*).

Stapes allograft

Stapes allografts are supplied for right or left reconstruction of the stapes in open mastoid cavity reconstruction and also can be used to advantage in ossicular tympanoplasty in the congenitally deformed middle ear.

  If there is no stapes arch, a stapes allograft may be put into position so that the footplate of the donor and recipient are in juxtaposition. However, if a portion of the patient's stapes crura remains, it can be removed with an argon laser so that the donor footplate fits directly against the patient's footplate. Also, the donor stapes footplate can be reduced in size, if necessary, with the argon laser. The stapes is then held in position with pledgets of Gelfoam soaked in 10% chloramphenicol and the posterior periosteal segment of the graft placed on to the area of the horizontal semicircular canal and into the mastoid cavity. The mastoid cavity may be lined with either fascia, rehydrated freeze-dried dura, or a muscle periosteal postauricular flap. The transplant and flaps are held in position with pledgets of Gelfoam soaked in 10% chloramphenicol.

Posterior osseous canal

Posterior osseous canal allografts may also be used to reconstruct small defects in the posterior osseous canal (for example, after some of the older atticotomy procedures).

Measuring instruments

Measuring instruments are necessary to determine the exact distance between the neck of the malleus and the head or the mobile footplate of the stapes. In addition, the measuring device serves as an instrument for lifting the malleus handle in order to obtain an accurate measurement.

The measuring instrument is similar to the House stapes prosthesis measuring device, but differs in that the metal post projection measures approximately 1 mm and can be used to lift up the malleus slightly as the surgeon is making the measurement between the head of the stapes or footplate and the neck of the malleus. The measuring devices are supplied in sizes from 2 to 5 mm; from 2 to 3 mm in 0.25 mm increments, and from 3 to 5 mm in 0.5 mm increments.

RESULTS

Any procedure for reconstruction of the middle ear transformer is difficult to evaluate except in the long term (5–8 years). Indications, techniques and modifications of alloplasts or allografts may alter results, making comparison difficult.

For example, from 1970 to 1975 all the otologic implants supplied by the Ear Transplant Unit of the Northern California Transplant Bank were processed and stored in tissue culture media with added antibiotics. Their shelf life was limited and the potential for transmission of disease or contamination existed. Hence, we changed to the ethylene oxide sterilization and freeze-drying method in 1976 and started supplying grafts processed in this manner to colleagues in 1978.

Over 2000 freeze-dried otologic transplants have been supplied by the Ear Transplant Unit of the Northern California Transplant Bank since 1976. There has been no evidence of transmission of infection by the transplant or any reactions to suggest rejection. Underlying ear disease, such as cholesteatoma, and abnormal Eustachian tube function affect graft acceptance. Extrusion, absorption and perforation have occurred in patients with poor Eustachian tube function and recurrent middle ear or mastoid infection. In a recent presentation to the American Otologic Society (Smith, 1982), 24 of 32 partial ossicular replacement allografts (75%) used in stable ears closed the air/bone gap within 10 dB. In the eight ears that did not have satisfactory functional hearing, this had become evident within one year and no further deterioration was noted up to 4 years. There was no evidence of extrusion or erosion.

Surgical conversion of the radical to the modified radical cavity using freeze-dried allograft material has been quite successful. Approximately 25% of the converted mastoid cavities do not develop postoperative Eustachian tube function; however, of the 75% that do develop an air-containing middle ear space, 50% closed the air/bone gap to within 10 dB, 30% closed within 20 dB, and 18% remained the same. Significant sensorineural loss was experienced by 2%.

The stapes was particularly useful in the conversion of the radical mastoid cavity to a modified radical cavity and also useful in the reconstruction of the congenitally anomalous middle ear transformer.

CAUSE OF FAILURE

In the ears that failed to close the air/bone gap to functional levels after insertion of the partial ossicular replacement allograft, there was either too great an angle between the neck of the malleus and stapes head or a distance in excess of 3.5 mm. Thus, it is essential that the surgeon determine accurately the distance between the head of the malleus and the stapes head and also calculate whether there is too large an angle between the stapes head and the malleus neck. At this point the surgeon must decide whether or not to reposition the tympanic membrane malleus unit, which will require slightly more removal of the posterior osseous canal than is removed at a stapedectomy procedure, in order to allow rotation of the malleus neck over the oval window. Then, in a second stage procedure 4 to 6 months later, a PORA can be placed between the malleus neck and stapes head. It will be obvious to the surgeon that in either the autograft or the allograft situation the tympanic membrane malleus unit can be positioned more advantageously over the oval window area.

CONCLUSION

Use of alloplasts in middle ear reconstruction (other than stapes replacement in otosclerosis) is suspect for long-term foreign body extrusion and poor functional results.

Otologic allografts (homografts) freeze-dried in ethylene oxide and sterilized offer an attractive alternative to the use of alloplasts and chemically fixed or heat-processed ossicular grafts for middle ear transformer reconstruction.

Further information

For additional information regarding the otologic transplants or measuring instruments, contact the Northern California Transplant Bank at the following address: Northern California Transplant Bank, 2340 Clay Street, PO Box 7999, San Francisco, CA 94115. Tel. (415) 922-3100.

References

DeSebastian, G. (1960) The replacement of portions of the ear ossicles with artificial substances. *Acta oto-rino-laringológica ibéro-americana*, **11**, 259–268

Guilford, F. R. (1965) Repositioning of the incus. *Laryngoscope*, **75**, 236–241

Glaninger, J (1964) Ossicular chain reconstruction. *Zeitschrift für Laryngologie, Rhinologie und Otologie*, **43**, 184–190

Hall, A. and Rytzner, C. (1957) Stapedectomy and autotransplantation of ossicles. *Acta Otolaryngologica*, **47**, 318–325

House, W. F., Patterson, M. and Lithicum, F. H., Jr. (1966) Incus homografts in chronic ear surgery. *Archives of Otolaryngology*, **84**, 148–153

Jansen, C. (1958) Über Radikaloperation und Tympanoplastik. *Stizungsber Fortbild, Arzetek*. obV, February 18

Kerr, A. G (1981) Protoplast and Plastipore. *Clinical Otolaryngology*, **6,** 187–192

Matte, (1901) Über Versuche mit Anheilung des Trommelfells an das Kopfchen des Steigbügels nach operative Behandlung chronischer Mittelöhreiterungen. *Archiv für Ohrenheilkunde*, **53,** 96–99

Rosomoff, H. L. (1959) Ethylene oxide sterilized, freeze-dried dura mater for the repair of pachymeningeal defects. *Journal of Neurosurgery*, **16,** 197

Shea, J. J. and Homsy, C. A. (1974) The use of Proplast TM in otologic surgery. *Laryngoscope*, **84,** 1835–1845

Shea, J. J. and Emmett, J. R. Jr (1978) Biocompatible ossicular implants. *Archives of Otolaryngology*, **104,** 191–196

Sheehy, J. L. (1965) Ossicular problems in tympanoplasty. *Archives of Otolaryngology*, **81,** 115–122

Sheehy, J. L. (1978) TORPs and PORPs in tympanoplasty. *Clinical Otolaryngology*, **3,** 451–454

Siedentop, K. H. and Brown, R. G. (1966) Type 3 polyethylene columella tympanoplasty. Long range review of 28 cases. *Archives of Otolaryngology*, **83,** 560–565

Smith, M. F. W. (1980) Freeze-dried otologic implants. *Journal of Otolaryngology*, **9,** 222–227

Smith, M. F. W. (1982) Lyophilized partial ossicular replacement allografts. *Annals of Otology, Rhinology and Laryngology* (in press)

Smyth, G. D. L. and Kerr, A. G. (1967) Homologous grafts for ossicular reconstruction in tympanoplasty. *Laryngoscope*, **77,** 330–336

Smyth, G. D. L. (1982) Five year report on PORPs and TORPs. *Otolaryngology, Head and Neck Surgery*, **90,** May/June, 343–346

Strauss, P. (1979) Vergleich von Ambossinterposition und Kuntstoffcolumella bei der tympanoplastie. *Zeitschrift für Laryngologie, Rhinologie und Otologie*, **58**(1), 15–22

5
Otosclerosis: an instruction course
Howard P. House and James L. Sheehy

TECHNIQUES

Personal experiences of Dr Howard House

In 1954 I was invited to New York by Dr Joseph Goldman, who was at that time Chairman of the Department at Mt Sinai Hospital, to see the new operation for otosclerosis by Dr Sam Rosen (1953). At that time, the procedure was considered new because it was not realized that it had been performed at the turn of the century.

I was impressed as Rosen elevated the tympanomeatal flap and exposed the middle ear through the transcanal approach under local anesthesia. (This approach was developed by Dr Julius Lempert for his tympanosympathectomy operation for tinnitus. I had not, however, had the privilege of seeing Lempert perform this particular operation.)

Through a hand-held otoscope Dr Rosen used a curved needle with which he carefully applied gentle pressure in a circular motion on the incus over the head of the stapes. This seemed to be adequate in a very minimally fixed stapes, and the patient would often hear immediately. If the stapes could not be mobilized by this maneuver, he applied the same gentle pressure directly on the head of the stapes, first in a superior-inferior motion and then in an anterior-posterior motion. Again, some would mobilize successfully. Fortunately, when the footplate was more than moderately fixed, the posterior or the anterior crus, or both, would fracture and these patients, if suitable, could then have the fenestration procedure at a later date.

After observing several of these operations, I visited a patient in whom Dr Rosen had mobilized the stapes some six months earlier and who had recovered his hearing.

On returning to Los Angeles with a set of instruments provided by Dr Rosen, I began first on temporal bones and later on patients undergoing fenestration surgery. I soon realized that, even with the ideal exposure of the stapes provided during the fenestration procedure, I could successfully mobilize the stapes without fracturing the crura in only one third of cases.

Rosen and many others began using small chisels directly on the anterior area of the fixed footplate. Others used needles to scrape through the anterior otosclerotic bone. Dr John Shea developed a small microdrill to drill through the otosclerotic region. I modified a dental pneumatic hammer, as used to put in amalgam fillings, to tap the otosclerotic region. About this time, Rosen began using a type of crochet needle to simply create an open hole in the footplate without attempting to mobilize the stapes. This was unsuccessful in restoring hearing and must have created a number of undetected fistulas.

These various attempts directly on the footplate bypassed the crura and therefore led to fewer operative failures due to crural fracture. Still, most of the cases refixed after six months or a year. Occasionally I still see patients whom I mobilized 25 years ago who are continuing to maintain closure of their bone–air gap. This, however, is an extremely rare occurrence.

Dr Ned Fowler, Chairman of the Department of Otolaryngology at Columbia University, New York, developed an anterior crurotomy procedure based on the theory that most otosclerotic fixation is anterior while the posterior half of the footplate is free of otosclerosis (Fowler, 1957). He came to Los Angeles to demonstrate the procedure, which to me seemed very logical, provided the anterior crus could be bisected without fracturing the posterior crus and the middle portion of the footplate could also be bisected by a sharp needle or chisel. This procedure seemed sound in theory but was very difficult to carry out in practice.

Dr John Shea, after finishing his residency at the Massachusetts Eye and Ear Infirmary, came to Los Angeles as a Fellow to spend time in otological surgery. At the time I was mobilizing stapes. In cases where the procedure was unsuccessful, I subsequently fenestrated the ear if the patient was suitable for this type of surgery. I recall Dr Shea asking me why not consider taking out the stapes in its entirety and inserting an artificial stapes. He felt that it would not be any more of a risk exposing the inner ear at the oval window than we were doing by making a fenestra nonovalis in the ampullated end of the horizontal canal. It was his feeling that if we sealed the oval window opening immediately we would protect the inner ear with minimal exposure.

Soon after this discussion Dr Shea returned to Memphis to begin practice. At the Triological meeting in Montreal a year later, I was moderating a panel discussion on stapes mobilization (House, 1958). John Shea showed me an artificial stapes which he had carved and designed to fit into the oval window with a means of attaching it to the incus. He had placed it in a patient and now showed me the preoperative and postoperative audiograms revealing complete closure of the bone–air gap. He asked to discuss this case at the close of the panel session and I arranged for him to do so. Needless to say, this young man's innovative presentation created considerable discussion. His effort was to revolutionize stapes surgery.

Stapedectomy is born

Events rapidly evolved and for several years (1956 to 1960) the technique changed quickly from mobilization to stapedectomy, with most of us using a vein graft to cover the window and connecting this with the incus by means of a polyethylene strut as advocated by Shea. This was the beginning of the end of the fenestration era. Today the only indication for fenestration surgery is a rare congenital aplasia involving the middle ear, which by its nature might require bypassing the middle ear in its entirety to get to the inner ear.

Within a few years it was realized that the polyethylene strut often tended to loosen, erode the long process of the incus and occasionally slip into the vestibule, especially on pressure changes, thereby resulting in acute vertigo and sensorineural hearing loss.

Use of the wire

Recognizing this problem of strut slippage and its disastrous results, Schuknecht (1960) used a wire which he attached to the incus and simply perforated the footplate. This did not result in much hearing change and he soon abandoned it in favor of total removal of the footplate, using a wire tied to fat to fill the oval window. This proved to be very successful and eliminated the strut problem. Others tied vein and Gelfoam which was attached to the wire and inserted it into the oval window.

Dr David Myers of Philadelphia began making a small hole in the footplate with a needle and inserting a 0.2 mm piston. This was unsuccessful in adequately closing the bone–air gap. Later, McGee introduced a 0.6 mm metal piston, which he and many others use today and which has proved very successful. Gilford of Houston developed a Teflon piston which also proved to be very successful. Smyth of Belfast and many others in the United States began using either the metal or the Teflon wire piston (either 0.4 or 0.6 mm in diameter) with very fine results. Some placed the piston over a tissue graft after total footplate removal and others simply made a hole directly in the fixed plate for insertion of the piston. I stayed with total stapedectomy for fear of fistula development with this type of piston technique.

1960 to 1977

Between 1960 and 1977, I covered the oval window with a compressed Gelfoam pad on which was placed the House double and later the single wire loop. As time went on, more and more surgeons were advocating tissue grafts of fascia or perichondrium as the covering membrane. My associate Sheehy discontinued using Gelfoam in 1968 and began using the wire loop over fascia. He was able to show us that this was superior to the Gelfoam pad covering (Sheehy and Perkins, 1976). After that time, our group gradually switched to using either fascia or perichondrium as a covering membrane, abandoning the Gelfoam pad technique.

During this time Dr Jack Hough of Oklahoma City developed a technique of bisecting the posterior crus at its attachment to the footplate but leaving it attached to the incus (Hough, 1960). He then bisected the anterior crus near the head of the stapes and removed the footplate in its entirety. A tissue graft was placed over the oval window, and the posterior crus was rotated anteriorly into position over the graft to connect the oval window area with the incus. This is a beautiful technique, which in the hands of Dr Hough achieves a fine result, but it is technically difficult for many others to duplicate.

Having realized that the small fenestra piston technique apparently did not cause more fistulas than total stapedectomy with tissue-covered oval windows, I adopted the piston technique in 1980 and am very pleased with the results.

My present technique

It has always seemed to me to be only logical that complications are less likely to occur with minimal inner ear exposure than with total removal of the footplate. Fortunately, however, there seems to be no clinical proof of this hypothesis.

For several years, in selected cases with a thin bluish footplate, I carried out fragmentation of the footplate, using a Gelfoam pad to cover the fragmented plate inserting the single wire loop into position. In these cases there was minimal perilymph escape and very little postoperative unsteadiness. Several revisions, however, were necessary to remove a scratching sound due to the wire rubbing on these fragments. Therefore, this technique was abandoned, even though refixation of the fragments was not a probability since the bluish footplate is cartilaginous in origin and has no osteogenic capability.

A few years ago Dr Rodney Perkins (1980) developed a laser technique for making the opening in the footplate to receive the piston. We acquired the equipment and this converted me from the total to the partial, small fenestra technique. A series of primary cases were treated using the argon laser, needles or a 0.7 mm cutting burr to make the opening in the footplate to receive the 0.6 mm Schuknecht Teflon piston. After using all three methods the results seemed to be equivalent.

The incision is made in the usual manner and the flap elevated. Great care must be taken to identify the annular ligament and to place the elevator posterior to the ligament as one elevates the inferior portion of the tympanic membrane. Superiorly the elevation is carried to make contact with the malleus neck. A curet is used to gain exposure sufficient to see the fallopian canal superiorly and the tip of the pyramidal process posteriorly. Care should be taken to avoid traumatizing the chorda tympani nerve. If it is traumatized or stretched to the point of a tear, it should be sectioned, as symptoms seem to persist longer if the nerve is stretched than if it is sectioned. As a matter of fact, I have had to revise several cases with prolonged taste disturbance to section the nerve in order to relieve the patient's symptoms.

A measurement is made from the external surface of the inferior end of the incus to the central portion of the footplate. This measurement averages 4.5 mm but may vary from 3.5 to 5.5 mm. The measurement is reduced by 0.25 mm if one calls for the Schuknecht Teflon piston, since Dr Schuknecht measures from the under-surface of the incus. Since the body of the long process approximates 1 mm, this provides 0.75 mm extension of the piston into the vestibule area.

A very sharp, straight, thin needle is used to puncture the footplate with a sudden insertion. If an inadvertent mobilization should occur without fracture of the crura, the entire stapes can often be removed intact without creating a vacuum reaction in the vestibule. If the crura fracture is simultaneous with mobilization of the footplate, the small opening then allows one to move the floating footplate when inserting an obtuse 45 degree angle needle in the opening and elevating the fragments or the entire footplate, as the case may be.

I consider the floating footplate to be the most difficult complication in stapes surgery. At times it is necessary to use a burr in the posterior inferior area of the promontory in order to obtain an opening into which to insert a needle to remove the floating footplate. If there is an otosclerotic overhang anteriorly and the footplate does not bisect with this maneuver, and the incus prevents an unimpeded view, it may be necessary to remove the incus in order to remove the overhang with a drill and then remove the floating plate. In this instance an incus replacement prosthesis from the malleus is needed (Sheehy, Nelson and House, 1979). If one uses an argon laser, this rather uncommon complication can often be avoided. If a total stapedectomy is necessary, fascia or perichondrium is then used to cover the oval window and a wire loop is inserted measuring 0.25 mm more than the measured length from the external surface of the incus to the footplate.

Usually the footplate remains fixed after the arch of the stapes crura has been removed. An opening of 0.7 mm is created in the footplate using the laser, a 45 degree angle hook or a 0.7 mm cutting burr. This burr may either be attached to an electric drill or may be hand-held. In the event of a solid or obliterated plate, a cutting burr is used to create the 0.7 mm opening. When fracturing the crural arch with a curved Rosen needle one must use a sudden motion and always direct it toward the promontory and never toward the facial nerve.

The Schuknecht Teflon piston is first inserted into the opening and then slipped over the incus and crimped. If the opening is larger than intended, an 0.8 mm piston may be inserted. At times the entire posterior half of the footplate is mobilized and may then be removed. When this occurs, a 1.0 mm Teflon piston is used. It appears that pistons of all three diameters (0.6, 0.8 and 1 mm) work equally well as far as hearing results and gap closure are concerned. After insertion and crimping of the piston, venous blood drawn at the start of the operation is placed into the oval window; this partially clotted blood acts as a seal. At this point the flap is replaced.

If one encounters a solid or obliterated plate or if there is a preoperative sensorineural hearing loss of 20 dB or more, sodium fluoride 25 mg to be taken daily for one year is routinely prescribed.

I have found this piston technique to give good results in terms of gap closure; very rarely has a sensorineural loss been observed, and the patients seem to have only very minimal, if any, unsteadiness following surgery, probably due to minimal trauma and minimal loss of perilymph. In conclusion, I hasten to say that those surgeons who have a technique that is working well in their hands, and whose results are equal to those being reported by others (90% total closure of the gap and less than 2% sensorineural loss), should stay with their technique. I firmly believe that the various techniques commonly used today by capable operators are giving equal results.

POSTOPERATIVE MANAGEMENT

Surgery is performed under local anesthesia with heavy premedication, and patients are returned to their room immediately following surgery. They are instructed to lie quietly in bed for a few hours and to request help from the nurse the first time they wish to leave the bed. Following that the patient is allowed to ambulate, if desired, but most have some dizziness on change of position and prefer to remain in bed.

Dimenhydrinate (Dramamine) is administered before meals and at bed time, by intramuscular injection if necessary. We administer perphenazine (Trilafon; Fentazin) 5 mg (once only) by injection should the patient have persistent vomiting, though this is rare. Sulfisoxazole (sulphafurazole; Gantrisin) 1 g four times a day is begun on admission to the hospital and continued for seven days postoperatively.

Patients are allowed to leave the hospital the morning after surgery. After removing the ear dressing and placing cotton in the meatus, we discuss with the patient postoperative instructions (of which he has received a copy at the preoperative visit). These are: do not blow the nose or allow water to enter the ear for three weeks. Obtain your medication (Gantrisin and Dramamine) from the nurse and follow the directions. You may return to normal activity, as desired, tomorrow. Any ear discharge should have subsided within a few days. Dizziness on change of position is not unusual for up to a week. I will see you in the office in three weeks. Call me should you have any problem. Air travel is allowed after two days.

Three to five days following surgery the otologist's surgery nurse telephones the patient to inquire about his or her progress. If necessary, the nurse will ask the surgeon to speak with the patient; this, however, is uncommon.

The first postoperative visit is scheduled for three weeks, at which time pure tone and speech hearing tests are performed, any crusts of blood are removed from the ear canal and the tympanic membrane is inspected for mobility. The patient is asked about dizziness (rare), taste disturbance or mouth dryness (present to a mild degree in about one fourth of patients, regardless of the chorda tympani management) and tinnitus (absent in 50%, less noticeable in 25% and unchanged in 25% of those who had tinnitus preoperatively). Many patients have a hollow feeling, a distorted sense of hearing, at this time. The patient is told that this is normal and will disappear by the second postoperative visit in four months.

At the four-month visit we perform pure tone and speech audiometry on both ears and discuss the possibility of surgery on the second ear, which we will perform six months or more after the first operation if the patient wishes. Additional follow-up hearing tests are recommended at one- to two-year intervals.

POSTOPERATIVE PROBLEMS

There are many transient postoperative symptoms which we anticipate and some problems (transient or otherwise) which are uncommon and are properly considered complications. These problems are taste disturbance, otitis externa, otitis media, dizziness, tympanic membrane perforations, facial paralysis, sensorineural hearing impairment and failure to gain hearing.

Taste disturbance and mouth dryness

Careful questioning at three weeks will reveal taste disturbance or mouth dryness, or both, in 25% of patients in whom the chorda tympani was not cut and in 45% of those in whom the chorda was cut. Less than half of these patients will mention the disturbance spontaneously. By the four-month visit only 15% still have symptoms, but only a third of these will mention the problem if not questioned.

Treatment of those rare patients who have a persisting problem with taste disturbance is for the most part symptomatic (gum chewing, water drinking, lifesavers), not scientific. Persistent symptoms are more common if the chorda tympani was stretched and in patients who have not obtained a good result from surgery or who have unilateral otosclerosis. If the chorda was left intact and disabling symptoms persist, re-elevation of the tympanomeatal flap and sectioning of the chorda tympani is often beneficial.

Generally speaking we will not perform surgery on the second ear if disabling symptoms persist. It is interesting that symptoms from the first ear may subside following surgery on the second ear, even in cases where chorda sectioning is required on the second ear.

Infection

All patients develop inflammatory reactions in the external auditory canal and middle ear following stapedectomy. The most common manifestation is the expected serous effusion of the middle ear. Routine use of prophylactic antibiotics usually prevents the inflammation from progressing to a frank infection.

Acute suppurative otitis externa or otitis media should be rare. When either occurs it is treated in the same way as in non-surgical cases.

Dizziness

We anticipate that all stapedectomy patients will have some dizziness for an hour or two on the day of surgery. Most will have some positional or postural vertigo on the first postoperative day, but rarely is this of a degree which requires continual hospitalization or even interferes significantly with walking. Three to five days following surgery (i.e. when the nurse telephones the patient) dizziness has usually subsided. By the end of three weeks it is a rare patient who mentions dizziness, but up to 10% will admit (upon questioning) to some postural vertigo. We reported a 2% incidence of non-disabling postural vertigo at four months and a 0.4% incidence of disabling vertigo; in all of these cases, however, the oval window had *not* been sealed with a tissue graft following total stapedectomy (Sheehy, Nelson and House, 1979).

But what about the patient who does have severe vertigo at some time during the first few weeks following stapedectomy? Should the ear be re-explored? Does the patient have an oval window fistula or granuloma? Will it heal spontaneously? How long should one wait to make a decision? We wish we had an answer to these questions, but we have not.

Severe vertigo occurring immediately after surgery and persisting for more than 12 hours is uncommon. When it occurs, the patient is kept in hospital and treated symptomatically. Severe vertigo may develop suddenly four to seven days following surgery and last for a day. Reassurance and symptomatic treatment are in order. Should the spontaneous vertigo persist longer we may prescribe vasodilators or prednisone, or both.

We do not recommend early revision (i.e. after one to two months), regardless of the symptoms, if the prosthesis is one that is securely attached to the incus (or malleus), as it should be. If there is a persistent balance disturbance which incapacitates the patient, we usually look for other contributing factors before re-exploring the ear. Remember that despite the fact that the dizziness followed surgery, multiple other factors may be responsible. We once had a patient with excellent postoperative hearing but episodic vertigo who was cured eventually by a high-protein, low-carbohydrate diet when it was discovered that she had severe reactive hypoglycemia which had undoubtedly existed prior to surgery without symptoms. Another patient with excellent postoperative hearing was cured of his persistent motion unsteadiness, which had lasted six months, by eliminating pork from the diet!

If the ear is re-explored because of a disabling balance disturbance, let us give you a word of advice: do not reopen the oval window unless you find a fistula or some other clear-cut explanation for the balance disturbance. There may be an inner ear problem, which is only made worse by opening the window. This worsening may result in a total sensorineural hearing loss (Sheehy, Nelson and House, 1981).

Tympanic membrane perforation

Perforation of the tympanic membrane following stapedectomy should be a rare occurrence in the absence of an acute otitis media if one pays attention to detail at the time of surgery.

Small tears of the tympanic membrane or flap occur at the annular margin in up to 1% of cases. Immediate repair by an undersurface graft of fascia, perichondrium or fat (from the lobule) or Gelfoam on the outer surface, or both, will almost always result in good healing.

Perforations occasionally occur due to a 'blow-out' of an old, thin, healed perforation. In these cases it is wise to reinforce the area with Gelfoam or tissue on the outer surface of the membrane at the end of surgery. Both will remain in place for a few weeks and prevent a blow-out, or facilitate healing should a perforation develop.

Should a central perforation be present at the three-week visit this will usually heal. Nonetheless, a paper patch is indicated. If the perforation is marginal, as it usually is, healing may not occur. We usually wait for four months before considering myringoplasty.

Facial paralysis

Facial paralysis is occasionally noted immediately following surgery due to the local anesthesia. This will resolve within hours. Should it not do so, and we have not encountered this, we would advise treatment with prednisone as for Bell's palsy.

Facial paralysis occurring 5 to 10 days after surgery is rare, but we do see this following both stapedectomy and tympanoplasty. If partial, as is usual, reassurance, vasodilators and eye protection are all that is indicated. If complete, the patient should be followed with electrical tests, as in Bell's palsy, and treated with prednisone.

Sensorineural hearing impairment

Sensorineural hearing impairment is the most serious postoperative stapedectomy complication and the patient must be made aware of this possibility, slight as it is, when surgery is first discussed. We tell our patients that there is a 2% chance of further hearing deterioration, to the point that an aid will not be usable, and a less than 1% chance of a total loss of hearing in the ear. Both are exaggerations, but the patient must not be lulled into a false sense of 'nothing can go wrong'.

A temporary sensorineural hearing impairment of 16 dB or more (or a discrimination impairment of 16% or more) has been detected in up to 5% of our tissue graft stapedectomy cases. This is usually noted at or before three weeks and has resolved by the end of four months without treatment.

A permanent sensorineural impairment of similar degree is detected in 2.6% of cases. Impairments of 30 dB (or a 30% discrimination) or more are noted in less than 1% of all stapedectomies with a tissue graft covering of the window. Total loss of hearing occurred in 0.4% of one series and 0.2% of another (Sheehy and Perkins, 1976). The three cases involved had Gelfoam used as a window covering, a technique no longer recommended.

Much of what has been said about the management of the dizzy patient applies here. We do not recommend early re-exploration of the ear with sensorineural impairment, but may explore it if there is dizziness, always remembering the advice given earlier, that is, not to open the window in a revision unless an obvious cause for the impairment is detected.

Failure to gain hearing

We anticipate that 90% or more of stapedectomy patients will have a postoperative conductive deficit (measured to the best bone conduction, preoperatively or postoperatively) of 10dB or less. In 96%, the deficit should be 15 dB or less. This leaves 4% with less than a satisfactory result. Should the ear be revised? Probably not, unless the deficit is 20 dB or more (Sheehy, Nelson and House, 1981).

Once again, the oval window should not be opened in a case with a postoperative balance disturbance or postoperative sensorineural impairment unless a fistula or a slipped or long prosthesis, that is, a possible cause for the inner ear symptom, can be identified. Finally, there is rarely an indication for a repeat drill-out of obliterative otosclerosis.

Acknowledgement

Work from the Otologic Medical Group, Inc., is supported by funds from the House Ear Institute, Los Angeles, an affiliate of the University of Southern California.

References

Fowler, E. P. (1957) Anterior crurotomy and mobilization of the ankyloid stapes footplate. *Acta Oto-Laryngologica*, **46**, 318–325

House, H. P. (1958) Symposium: stapes mobilization two years later. *Laryngoscope*, **68**, 1403–1441

Hough, J. V. D. (1960) Partial stapedectomy. *Annals of Otology, Rhinology and Laryngology*, **69**, 571–580

Perkins, R. C. (1980) Laser stapedectomy for otosclerosis. *Laryngoscope*, **90**, 228–240

Rosen, S. (1953) Mobilization of the stapes to restore hearing in otosclerosis. *New York Journal of Medicine*, **53**, 2650–2657

Schuknecht, H. F. (1960) The metal prosthesis for stapes ankylosis. *American Medical Association Archives of Otolaryngology*, **71**, 287–291

Sheehy, J. L., Nelson, R. A. and House, H. P. (1979) Stapes surgery at the Otologic Medical Group. *American Journal of Otology*, **1**, 22–26

Sheehy, J. L., Nelson, R. A. and House, H. P. (1981) Revision stapedectomy: a review of 258 cases. *Laryngoscope*, **91**, 43–51

Sheehy, J. L. and Perkins, J. H. (1976) Stapedectomy: Gelfoam compared with tissue grafts. *Laryngoscope*, **86**, 436–444

6
Management of obliterative otosclerosis
Ronald E. Gristwood

DEFINITION

Obliterative otosclerosis refers to a massive otosclerotic focus which fills in and obliterates the oval window niche. There are wide geographical variations in the prevalence of this condition (Gristwood, 1966b). In Germany, Plester found obliterative otosclerosis in 2.3% of 1000 consecutive patients. In Los Angeles, USA, House encountered it in 1.2%of 800 primary cases of stapes surgery. By contrast, in South Australia, Gristwood and Venables (1975) discovered obliteration of the oval window niche in 11.2% of 1000 consecutive patients who underwent stapes surgery.

CLASSIFICATION

There are three classes of obliterated footplate (*Figure 6.1*), each requiring similar surgical management.

(1) *In the truly obliterated footplate*, the stapes footplate is greatly thickened and diffusely replaced by a massive otosclerotic focus which fills in the oval window niche in varying degrees. The rim of the footplate cannot be identified because there is no delineation to indicate the margin of the window. The stapedial crura are often partially, but rarely completely, buried in the proliferation of otosclerotic bone. It is not possible to remove the thickened footplate discretely from the oval window niche in these cases. The otosclerotic bone varies in hardness and in thickness (from 0.5 to 2.5 mm), and tedious use of micropicks or microburr within the oval window area is needed to create an opening into the vestibule of the labyrinth. The prevalence of this variant in South Australia is 6.1%.
(2) *The solid partially obliterated footplate* is diffusely and greatly thickened, but a rim of delineation, which is often spurious, can be seen over a small segment

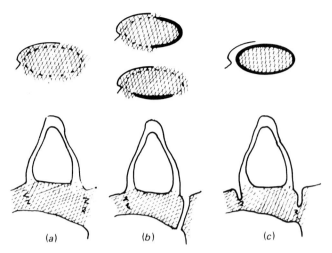

Figure 6.1 Diagram illustrating the three variants of the obliterated oval window niche. (*a*) Truly obliterated footplate; (*b*) partially obliterated footplate in which the limited segment of delineation may be polar or adjacent to the promontory; (*c*) spuriously delineated footplate. (From Gristwood and Venables, 1975, courtesy of the Editor and Publishers, *Journal of Laryngology and Otology*)

(25–50%) of its circumference, the remainder of the margin being obliterated. The segment of delineation may be polar or adjacent to the promontory at the lower margin of the window. (Prevalence in South Australia 4.6%.)

(3) *The solid spuriously delineated footplate* has a complete gutter of delineation surrounding what appears to be a thick solid footplate. The spurious nature of the delineation is only revealed when attempts to bisect and remove either half of the stapedial footplate fail because of deeper obliteration. (Prevalence in South Australia 0.5%.)

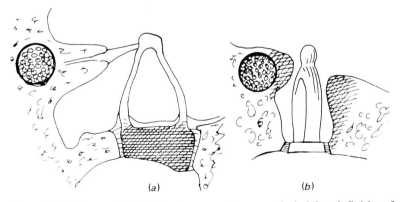

Figure 6.2 Diagram illustrating two conditions excluded by definition from the case of obliterative otosclerosis. (*a*) Solid delineated, 'thick biscuit' or 'rice-grain' footplate; (*b*) oval window niche narrowed by exostoses of promontory and facial canal. (From Gristwood and Venables, 1975, courtesy of the Editor and Publishers, *Journal of Laryngology and Otology*)

Conditions to be distinguished from obliterative otosclerosis

The three variants of the obliterated footplate described above should be clearly distinguished from two other conditions which are sometimes erroneously called obliterative otosclerosis. These are the *solid delineated footplate* and the *narrowed oval window niche (Figure 6.2)*.

The solid delineated footplate (also called the 'thick biscuit' or 'rice-grain' footplate) is diffusely and greatly thickened but retains a clearly delineated rim and an intact annular ligament so that surgical extraction of the footplate can be accomplished leaving a well-defined smooth edge to the oval window frame. The solid footplate is often tightly wedged in the oval window, but in some cases where fixation is less secure special care must be taken during operation if inadvertent mobilization and a floating footplate is to be prevented. Rarely is the gutter of delineation surrounding a solid footplate found to be spurious. (Prevalence in South Australia 12.5%.)

The narrowed oval window niche is the result of otosclerotic foci around the oval window niche forming exostoses which substantially overlap and narrow the niche. The narrow niche does not come under the definition of obliterative otosclerosis. The pathological classification of a case is determined by the degree of involvement of the footplate in the otosclerotic lesion. A narrow niche may be seen with a relatively thin footplate or with a severely thickened footplate. In South Australia, the oval window niche was seen to be narrowed to less than 0.8 mm in 4.1% of cases of otosclerosis, but a slit-like niche was seen in only 0.3%.

PREOPERATIVE IDENTIFICATION OF OBLITERATIVE OTOSCLEROSIS

The question posed is whether the patient with obliterative otosclerosis can be identified with any certainty before operation. The age at onset of hearing loss is an important indicator of this condition (Gristwood, 1966a). An early age of onset of hearing impairment, i.e. during the period of skeletal growth, dramatically increases the chance of contracting a fulminating lesion with severe and diffuse involvement of the stapes footplate or obliteration of the oval window niche (Gristwood and Venables, 1982). Of 279 otosclerotic patients in South Australia with onset of deafness before the age of 20 years, 132 (47.3%) had major footplate pathology at the time of operation. On the other hand, a late age of onset (30 years and upwards) of clinical otosclerosis tends to be associated with lesions limited to the anterior pole of the footplate.

Tympanometry in otosclerosis shows that middle ear pressures are usually atmospheric and that a wide range of compliance values is possible. Morrison (1979) considers that if the compliance variation is greater than $0.6\,cm^3$, it is highly probable that the fixed stapes footplate will be thin, while if the compliance variation is less than $0.2\,cm^3$, there is a reasonable likelihood of encountering a thick or obliterated footplate. In a smaller pilot study, the author was unable to confirm that small values of compliance variation (below $0.2\,cm^3$) were helpful in prediction, because the proportion of low compliance values was the same in both the thin and the thick footplate groups.

The patient with an obliterated footplate cannot be identified from a considera-tion of routine audiometric findings such as the air and bone conduction thresholds or the preoperative bone/air gap. It has been observed that the obliterated footplate is rarely encountered in unilateral stapedial otosclerosis.

SURGICAL MANAGEMENT

The massive otosclerotic focus, filling in and obliterating the oval window niche, was an ominous finding for those otologists who encountered it during stapes surgery in the early 1960s. Attempts to drill out the oval window were accompanied by an incidence of about 10% of severe cochlear deafness (Guilford, 1963; Schuknecht, 1963; Shea, 1963b), and there was a tendency of the bone to regrow with reclosure of the window in 50% of the cases (Bellucci, 1978; House, 1962).

Because of the poor results accruing from surgery on the oval window in this type of case, several otologists (Guilford, 1963; Hall, 1963; Hough, 1963; Sullivan, 1963; Walsh, 1965; Cody, Hallberg and Simonton, 1967), some even as late as 1967, were of the opinion that the obliterated footplate was a contraindication to surgery of the oval window and that classical fenestration of the lateral semicircular canal was the safest and most successful procedure if the patient had adequate cochlear reserve.

Despite the discouraging difficulties and daunting experiences, some otologists (Shea, 1963b; Sooy, Owens and Theurer, 1964a, b; Willis, 1964) persisted in an oval window approach. In 1962, Shea introduced his Teflon piston technique, which was a less traumatic operation and used a small fenestra into the vestibule (Shea, 1962, 1963a). The early success rates of this method encouraged other workers (McGee, 1965; Gristwood, 1966b, 1970; Ford *et al.* 1971) to use piston techniques for obliterative otosclerosis with similarly gratifying results in the short term (Shea, 1969).

At the possible risk of oversimplification, one might say that the problem of the obliterated oval window has been largely solved by the use of solid piston-shaped prosthetic devices made of Teflon, stainless steel or Teflon steel wire. The technique of the piston operation in obliterative otosclerosis, the difficulties and complications arising during and after surgery, and the short- and long-term hearing results achieved in 140 patients are described and discussed below.

The piston technique

The safest and least traumatic operation in obliterative otosclerosis is one in which an opening of only 1 mm in diameter is carefully created in the centre of the bone filling in the oval window niche. The presence of a piston placed within this opening precludes encroachment of the space it occupies by any further bone growth. Moreover, the intrusion medially of the tip of the piston into the perilymph-filled vestibule some 0.25 to 0.5 mm beyond the otosclerotic focus makes it unlikely that any proliferation of new bone will grow deep to the piston to immobilize it. Experience, time and careful follow-up studies have supported these theoretical considerations.

Drill-out procedures with extensive burring to develop an oval window of normal dimensions (2 × 3 mm) carry a high risk of surgical trauma to the inner ear and are therefore best avoided.

The main points of the surgical technique are considered briefly below.

Anaesthesia

The operation can be carried out under local or general anaesthesia according to the preferences of surgeon and patient. In Australia and Great Britain most patients desire a general anaesthetic.

The two essentials for success in any microsurgical procedure on the middle ear are haemostasis and immobility (Hall and Millar, 1950). A general anaesthetic, while ensuring immobility of the patient, may not give the relatively bloodless operative field required, and straining or coughing may be induced when the head is moved on the endotracheal tube at the completion of the procedure, thus producing displacment of tissue seals and engendering potential fistula formation at the oval window.

The services of a skilled anaesthetist who is experienced in anaesthesia for this type of surgery are mandatory if conditions safe for the patient and suitable for the surgeon are to be obtained.

General anaesthesia may be combined with (a) hypotensive agents or (b) haemostatic injection of adrenaline solution to produce bloodless conditions for surgery.

Haemostasis

The patient is placed on the operating table with the ear to be operated on uppermost. Haemostasis is assisted by careful positioning of the patient's head and body to provide for free venous return through the neck. Tilting of the table so that the head is higher than the trunk and lower limbs reduces venous pressure in the operative field. It is only by use of a correctly applied haemostatic injection (Gristwood, 1969) that intense vasoconstriction and excellent haemostasis can be achieved with near-certainty in the operation area for periods of up to 2 hours.

HAEMOSTATIC SOLUTION

The adult patient receives a haemostatic injection of 5.0 to 7.5 ml of freshly prepared 1% lignocaine (lidocaine) and 1 in 30 000 adrenaline (0.17 to 0.25 mg adrenaline) injected into the site of the incision and around the external auditory canal either before or after anaesthesia is induced. Minimal discomfort is experienced by the sedated conscious patient during the injection if a 26 gauge, 5 cm long needle is used attached to a 10 ml Luer-lok syringe. An aspiration test must be made before injection to guard against inadvertent intravascular administration, and, ideally, 15 min should elapse before any incision is commenced.

In stapedectomy, four sites are routinely injected.

(1) The needle is directed forwards and slightly upwards from a point in the postauricular sulcus to reach the region between the root of the helix and tragus a few millimetres above the entrance to the auditory canal and superficial to the deep fascia covering temporalis muscle. Initially, 2 to 3 ml of solution are deposited to produce localized swelling and blanching of skin in this area (effect on superficial temporal vessels and auriculotemporal nerves).

(2) From the same point in the retro-auricular sulcus, the needle is directed downwards and forwards over the mastoid tip to reach below the concha and membranous meatus, and 1 to 2 ml of solution is injected during withdrawal over the mastoid tip (effect on posterior auricular vessels, great auricular nerve and possibly auricular branch of vagus).

(3) The needle is placed within the auditory meatus and passed downwards and medially to pierce forcibly the cartilage of the membranous meatus near its union with the bony meatus. After preliminary aspiration, 1.5 ml of solution is injected deep to the parotid gland and above the posterior belly of the digastric muscle (effect on posterior auricular artery, its stylomastoid branch, the deep auricular artery and the facial nerve – temporary paresis in approximately 20% of cases).

(4) The needle is placed within the auditory meatus and directed upwards and medially to strike the roof of the bony canal. An injection of 0.5 ml is made subperiosteally to blanch the vascular strip.

PRECAUTIONS

It is known that (a) the injection of adrenaline can produce cardiac arrhythmias in animals and in man if a large enough dose is given; (b) the dose of adrenaline required to produce cardiac arrhythmias is less in patients anaesthetized with cyclopropane, trichloroethylene or halothane than in those anaesthetized with nitrous oxide or in the absence of general anaesthesia; (c) the intravenous dose of adrenaline required to produce arrhythmias is much smaller than the intramuscular or subcutaneous dose; and (d) hypercarbia and/or hypoxia appear to be factors which contribute to the production of cardiac arrhythmias (Katz and Katz, 1966).

Therefore, when general anaesthesia is required, a skilled anaesthetist is essential to ensure safe conditions for the patient in the presence of injected adrenaline. The surgeon, for his part, must avoid intravenous injection of adrenaline by doing an aspiration test before *every* injection. Subject to these precautions, the use of adrenaline by injection as outlined for local haemostasis is safe. No untoward incidents have occurred in a series of over 3000 operations with general anaesthesia using this haemostatic injection technique.

Preparation of outer ear and external auditory canal

Before the ear is prepared, the head is shaved to remove an area of hair extending approximately 2 cm in all directions from the rim of the pinna. The outer ear and its surroundings are then cleansed with a suitable antiseptic solution such as povidone-iodine. The skin is dried, operative drapes are applied and a plastic adhesive sheet is placed over the head and pressed against the skin to ensure that the drape adheres properly. The nurse and the surgeon should carefully remove all powder from their gloves by washing the gloved hands in warm water. Any wax, debris or antiseptic in the ear canal is removed by irrigation with Ringer's solution using a fine suction tip and the microscope.

Adequate exposure

The customary approach is transmeatal, using the largest size of speculum which can be inserted into the external auditory canal, where it is fixed in position with the speculum holder. Since 1963, the routine use of a small endaural incision (after Heermann and Plester) has allowed greatly improved access to the tympanum. Two small endaural retractors are placed perpendicularly to each other in the introitus of the external meatus to give the necessary exposure. This allows bimanual instrumentation within the meatus and offers ready access to connective tissue, which can be excised from the lips of the endaural incision or from temporalis fascia.

A rectangular tympanomeatal skin flap, about 8 to 10 mm long, is elevated from the underlying bone of the posterior canal wall using a microdissector and suction simultaneously. The fibrous tympanic annulus is identified, freed from the tympanic sulcus and lifted forwards to fold the posterior part of the tympanic membrane and skin flap over the anterior part of the tympanic membrane.

The chorda tympani nerve is preserved whenever possible and displaced anteriorly; nevertheless, it was found necessary to section it in about 25% of the obliterative cases in order to improve access.

Adequate surgical exposure of the oval window niche necessitates, in almost every case, removal of sufficient bone (about 1 or 2 mm) of the postero-superior margin of the tympanic ring with a sharp curette. Exposure is satisfactory when the whole oval window niche with the stapes, the tympanic portion of the facial canal above and the pyramid behind are clearly in view.

Inspection of tympanum

Fixation of the stapes is tested and confirmed by palpation. The incudostapedial joint is then separated and mobility of the malleus and incus is demonstrated. At this point the extent of footplate involvement in the otosclerotic lesion is estimated under higher magnification, the round window niche is examined for narrowing or occlusion by otosclerosis, and the facial canal is inspected for areas of dehiscence which are soft on palpation or bulging slightly. The stapedius tendon is divided close to its exit from the pyramid and the crural arch is fractured by displacing it towards the promontory and then removed.

Removal of mucoperiosteum

In otosclerosis the mucoperiosteum overlying the footplate and lining the walls of the oval window niche varies greatly in thickness and vascularity. In this series of 140 cases of obliterative otosclerosis the mucosa over the footplate was thin, delicate and avascular in approximately 50%, thick and avascular in 20%, and thickened and vascular in 30%. The mucoperiosteum is incised and elevated from the oval window area. Any bleeding is controlled by application of a small pledget of gelatin sponge moistened with a solution of 1 in 1000 adrenaline.

Opening into the vestibule

The hardness of the bone obliterating the oval window niche is tested by a Heermann micropick. It seems not unreasonable to equate hardness with the relatively mature, mineralized mosaic bone of healed, inactive otosclerosis, and softness with the immature, poorly mineralized, woven structure of fibrous bone seen in active otosclerosis. The bone was found to be soft in 25% and hard in 75% of our cases.

Where the bone of the obliterated footplate is soft and friable a micropick is carefully used to ream out bone between the two crural stumps so as to create an opening about 1 mm in diameter into the vestibule. Particular care must be taken during this procedure to ensure that the saccule and utricle do not come into contact with instruments or fragments of bone.

When the bone in the window is relatively hard a microdrill with an angled handpiece and a geared steel penetrator burr (Richards Manufacturing Company, Catalogue No. 13-0460) is needed. Suitable alternatives are a steel cutting burr or a diamond-paste burr with a diameter of 1 mm. The microdrill is used intermittently, gently and fairly slowly to enable a bore hole 1 mm in diameter to be created without damage to inner ear structures or facial nerve. Suction and irrigation can be used only intermittently at intervals when the drill is laid aside. When the bone in the depth of the bore attains the blue stage of thinness the drill is discarded and the final disc of bone is punctured and removed by a microhook. Before the blue stage of thinness is achieved one can usually notice 'sweating' of the bone due to seepage of perilymph through it. During the drilling procedure it has been found important to ensure that the shank of the burr is almost in contact with the long process of the incus so that an optimal angle of drill shaft is obtained for the piston in relation to its attachment to the incus (*Figure 6.3*).

A policy of deliberate saucerization of the oval window niche has not been found necessary for piston cases. Any promontory overhang narrowing the niche has to be taken down carefully with the diamond burr. The thickness of the bone of the obliterated footplate can be measured by noting the relation of the shoulder of the burr to the depth of drilling. Approximately a quarter of the obliterated cases had a bone thickness of between 0.5 and 0.9 mm, two thirds had a bone thickness of between 1 and 1.9 mm, and the remaining tenth had a bone thickness of 2 mm or greater.

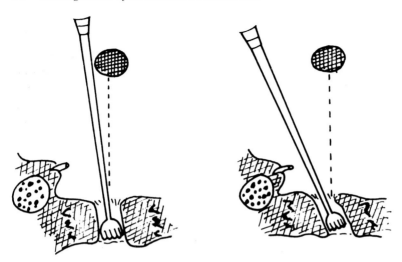

Figure 6.3 Drilling axis. Diagram showing favourable (left) and unfavourable (right) axis of drilling in relation to the attachment of piston to incus (From Gristwood and Venables, 1975, courtesy of the Editor and Publishers, *Journal of Laryngology and Otology*)

The solid spuriously delineated footplate is fortunately rare, because the presence of delineation suggests a method of surgical technique that is inappropriate for the obliterated oval window. The spurious nature of the delineation is only revealed after the footplate has been bisected coronally, and attempts to remove either half of the footplate fail because of obliteration deeper in. Faced with this situation the surgeon has no alternative but to use microhooks in an attempt to create an opening large enough in the bisecting channel to allow insertion of a piston. If the bone is hard the procedure can be extremely tedious. The drill cannot be safely used in the circumstance of the open vestibule.

Selection of piston

In many cases of obliteration of the oval window niche by a massive otosclerotic lesion there is some degree of bulging of the footplate focus into the labyrinthine vestibule. Schuknecht's manual of *Stapedectomy* (1971) contains several photo-micrographs illustrating this feature of extension of the disease beyond the usual footplate level. The practical importance of being aware of this medial protrusion of the lesion is that a fractionally longer piston prosthesis is required than for the more usual thin footplate to ensure long-term hearing improvement after stapedectomy. The piston has to be sufficiently long to extend into the vestibule beyond the otosclerosis focus so that further bony growth and immobilization is made less likely. Usually a piston 0.5 mm longer than the distance measured between the medial aspect of the long process of incus and the vestibule has been selected, up to a maximum length of 5 mm. It is perhaps worth emphasizing that 56 of the 140 piston cases discussed in this chapter had a prosthesis 4.75 to 5.0 mm in length (measured from the medial aspect of the incus). In none of these cases, followed up for periods of 7 to 10 years, has immobilization of a piston by new bone growth occurred. In one patient persistent ataxia after operation was attributable to excessive piston length.

Of two piston diameters (0.8 and 0.6 mm), the slimmer version was used in 80% of the cases, and is now preferred for all obliterated footplates. Teflon and wire Teflon types of prosthesis were distributed equally throughout the cases, the Teflon piston being used almost exclusively before October 1966 and the wire Teflon piston after that. The prosthesis is inserted into the vestibule and its ring end (or wire hook) is gently placed over the long process of the incus. Careful positioning and crimping of the wire or Teflon loop is required to ensure perfect contact with the incus and thus ideal conditions for transmission (*Figure 6.4*). The wire Teflon

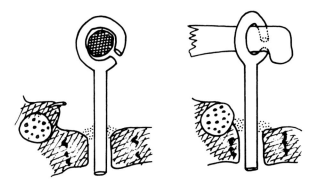

Figure 6.4 Teflon piston *in situ*. Diagram illustrating the correct placement and attachment of the Teflon piston after drill-out of obliterated oval window. (From Gristwood and Venables, 1975, courtesy of the Editor and Publishers, *Journal of Laryngology and Otology*)

has an advantage over the Teflon in that the wire can be slightly angulated when necessary to adapt to difficult anatomical situations. After crimping, the piston should be most gently palpated to demonstrate its mobility within the oval window opening.

Seal for oval window

All cases of piston operation have a temporary perilymphatic fistula at the oval window until a new endosteal membrane forms over the deep intralabyrinthine aspect of the piston. Strips of gelatin sponge or pieces of soft connective tissue placed as a collar around the piston at its entrance into the drill hole are designed to seal this fistula until regeneration of endosteum has occurred. Personal preference is now for a soft connective tissue seal, although no instance of recurrent or late fistula has been noted in any case of obliterated oval window in which a piston device has been used with a gelatin sponge seal.

Closure

Lastly, the chorda tympani nerve is replaced, the tympanomeatal skin flap is folded back into position against the posterior canal wall and splinted by small pledgets of moist gelatin sponge, and the endaural incision is closed with three interrupted sutures of silk or nylon.

Antibiotic cover

Wound infection is exceptional after the stapedectomy operation, but, because the labyrinth has been opened, many surgeons prefer to give a prophylactic course of an antibiotic in the hope of preventing a possible infection which could have disastrous consequences for hearing were the labyrinth to become involved. The problems with antibiotic prophylaxis are, as various studies have shown, that the risk of acquiring an infection is not reduced, that wound infection can be caused by a number of different organisms which may not be sensitive to the antibiotic prescribed and that, if infection follows, it may be due to an organism resistant to the drug given and therefore more difficult to treat (Sleigh, 1974).

It is the author's practice to give a single intramuscular injection of benzyl penicillin 600 mg at the end of the operative procedure, provided there is no known hypersensitivity. There have been no cases of postoperative wound infection or of otitis media in the early postoperative period in 1500 consecutive stapedectomy procedures.

Many prefer to give trimethoprim with sulphamethoxazole (Bactrim, Septrin), one tablet by mouth twice daily for a period of five days.

Postoperative care

The postoperative management of the obliterative case differs in no way from that of the uncomplicated stapedectomy. The patient is confined to bed for the first 24 hours postoperatively, with the operated ear uppermost and the head on one or two pillows. Toilet privileges and gentle walking activities are then permitted if there is no postural vertigo. Nose blowing and sneezing are prohibited. Endaural sutures are removed on the third or fourth postoperative day, at which time the patient is allowed home. The gelatin sponge packing is removed from the ear between the seventh and tenth day, and a dressing of half-inch ribbon gauze impregnated with antibiotic corticosteroid ointment is inserted for a further 5 days if healing of incisions is not complete.

Audiometric assessments are arranged at 1, 3, 6 and 12 months postoperatively.

POSTOPERATIVE REVIEW OF PATIENTS

The importance of adequate follow-up of patients can hardly be over-emphasized if one is to confirm or refute that the long-term results of surgical treatment are quite as satisfactory as those in the short term, or if any complications that ensue are to be observed and rectified. Since 1965, all patients suitable for stapes surgery have been asked to agree to participate in a 10-year programme of audiological assessments at 1, 2, 3, 5, 7 and 10 years after operation. This psychological preparation, together with determined efforts at follow-up, has successfully reduced the number of patients who are not available for review at various intervals after surgery (*Table 6.1*).

Table 6.1 Follow-up of 140 cases of obliterative otosclerosis

	3 Months	1 Year	3 Years	5 Years	7 Years	10 Years
Patients traced	140 (100%)	133 (95%)	122 (87.1%)	114 (81.4%)	94 (67.1%)	61/125 (48.8%)*
Patients dead	none	none	1 (0.8%)	5 (3.6%)	9 (6.4%)	9 (7.2%)
Patients untraced	none	7 (5.0%)	17 (12.1%)	21 (15.0%)	37 (26.5%)	55 (44.0%)

* Fifteen cases not included as their potential follow-up of 10 years had not been reached when the analysis was performed.

SURGICAL COMPLICATIONS AND FAILURES

Various complications have been observed at, or following, surgery in these 140 obliterative cases.

(1) *Massive multiple exostoses of bony external auditory canal* (1 case). These may necessitate a two-stage procedure if an intact tympanomeatal flap cannot be developed and maintained.
(2) *Obliteration of the round window niche* (2 cases). Complete obliteration of the round window niche is rare, although narrowing is not uncommon. Only 2 patients in this series, 1 male and 1 female, had total obliteration of the round window niche, the site of which could be seen as a mere dimple on the promontory. Both patients had greatly and diffusely thickened footplates (one obliterated and one delineated), and both had profound loss of hearing; bone conduction thresholds were not measurable in either patient. Neither case achieved any hearing improvement after surgery.
(3) *Obliteration of the labyrinthine vestibule* (1 case). Massive proliferation of the otosclerotic focus with invasion and obliteration of the vestibule is a most singular phenomenon, and fortunately so, because it defies all possibility of remedy apart, perhaps, from Plester's (1970, 1971) method of creating a promontorial window directly into the scala vestibuli. Only one case of otosclerotic obliteration of the labyrinthine vestibule has been encountered in the last 20 years. This was a young male of 18 years with rapidly progressive bilateral impairment of hearing from the age of 10 years who had been subjected to a classical fenestration of his right ear at the age of 12, and a vein graft stapedectomy of his left ear at the age of 14, neither procedure giving

benefit. The thresholds of hearing for air and bone conduction were not recordable at the maximum output of the audiometer. Revision surgery of his left ear revealed a patent round window niche, and obliteration of the oval window and cavity of vestibule by soft vascular spongy bone.

(4) *Inadvertent entry of burr into vestibule* (2 cases). In one patient the mishap was not associated with turbulence of perilymph, and a good functional result was obtained. In the second patient the drill was used to a depth of 2 mm when the burr entered the vestibule. Marked turbidity of perilymph was noted. Although the patient had a gain of hearing of 25 dB, maintained over 5 years, there was depreciation of bone conduction thresholds by 20 dB and depression of word discrimination scores to less than 20%.

(5) *Loss of bone fragments into vestibule* (6 cases). In 6 patients a small bony disc or fragment disappeared into the vestibule after drilling, one disc remaining hinged and five sinking slowly out of sight. No attempt was made to retrieve these small particles of bone, all of which were less than 1 mm in diameter. All cases had a satisfactory gain of hearing. Five cases were asymptomatic, but one complained of brief episodes of postural vertigo for three months, after which the symptom settled down.

(6) *Primary cochlear failure* (1 case). One case referred to under (4) above had partial cochlear failure due to the trauma of drilling.

(7) *Absence of hearing gain* (10 cases). Ten patients failed to achieve any significant gain of hearing in the early postoperative period. These were all patients with far-advanced otosclerosis in which the bone conduction threshold was not measurable on a standard clinical audiometer and the air conduction level was in excess of 95 dB ISO (Sheehy, 1964).

There were 22 cases of profound deafness in the present group of cases of obliterative otosclerosis, and 12 have achieved and maintained some gain of hearing and have had benefit from an insert hearing aid in the treated ear. Such cases of profound deafness should, therefore, be given an opportunity by surgery to restore what little is possible for them within the limits of their severely impaired sensorineural function. The diagnostic points (besides the history of progressive hearing loss with paracusis Willisii in the early stages and, perhaps, a familial history of deafness) are a quiet well modulated voice and often a still-perceived negative Rinne response to strongly vibrating tuning forks of C^1, C^2, and C^3.

(8) *Delayed cochlear failure* (2 cases). One case, a female aged 44 years, experienced sudden hearing loss with severe tinnitus at 5 months after surgery. The cause remains obscure, since there was no evidence of perilymph fistula at the oval window when the middle ear was explored.

The second case, a female aged 59 years, had maintained excellent hearing at the 22 dB level with normal word discrimination for 6 years after surgery. She then had a 5-month course of daily intramuscular streptomycin for active pulmonary tuberculosis, following which the hearing slowly deteriorated (without tinnitus) in the operated ear. At 9 years postoperatively she has near normal hearing up to 500 Hz, with a steep sensory loss above that frequency, and poor word discrimination of 64%.

(9) *Delayed conductive loss* (4 cases). These occurred at 5, 24 (2 cases) and 30 months after surgery, 3 cases being due to necrosis of the distal third of the long process of the incus, and 1 due to the wire of a Teflon wire piston becoming detached from the incus. In 2 cases, pressure necrosis had resulted from use of the original model of Teflon piston (slit at vertex of ring) on an incus with a slightly thicker long process than usual. In the third case, the ring of the Teflon prosthesis had slipped off an incus shaft already attenuated by erosion at the time of the original surgery. In all 4 cases the piston had extruded from the oval window which was filled in by soft connective tissue. There was no case of bony reclosure of the drill hole. The wire Teflon piston would appear to be preferable for those cases in which the incus shaft has abnormal dimensions, because a more accurate adjustment of prosthesis to incus is then possible by appropriate crimping of the wire loop.

(10) *Positional vertigo and persistent imbalance* (2 cases). In 1 patient, persistent ataxia after operation was attributable to excessive length of the prosthesis. The middle ear was explored, the piston (5 × 0.6 mm) extracted and a shorter one re-inserted with complete disappearance of the imbalance. In another patient, postural vertigo persisted for 3 months after operation at which a tiny disc of bone fell into the vestibule. The symptom cleared up spontaneously.

(11) *Perilymphatic fistula at oval window*. No fistula has been noted at exploratory tympanotomy of 5 cases whose hearing deteriorated (1 cochlear and 4 conductive).

(12) *Bony reclosure of the window*. This has not been observed in any case of obliterative otosclerosis for which a piston technique was used and the case followed up for 7 to 10 years.

(13) *Facial paralysis* (2 cases). This is fortunately a rare complication of stapes surgery, and has occurred in 3 cases in 1500 consecutive stapes operations. All were temporary and 2 of them occurred in obliterated cases. In one case, in which the facial paralysis had a delayed onset (seven days postoperatively) and a duration of 35 days, complete recovery took place.

The second case was of immediate onset in a male aged 44 years whose oval window niche was covered by a greatly thickened mucoperiosteum during removal of which the completely exposed facial nerve was lifted and slightly stretched on the point of a needle. Recovery of movement of the lower half of the face was complete within 3½ months, but recovery of frontalis movement remains only partial.

The risk of damaging the facial nerve during drilling of the obliterated oval window is considerable unless great care is taken to ensure accurate placement of the burr and avoidance of overheating.

(14) *Malleo-vestibulopexy* (1 case). The connection of a prosthesis from the malleus handle to the vestibule was necessary in 1 female patient of 28 years whose incus long process was a mere stump. A subperiosteal tunnel was therefore created over the upper half of the malleus handle to allow insertion of a Teflon piston (4.5 × 0.6 mm). The long-term audiometric result of this case at 7 years postoperatively is shown in *Figure 6.5*. The bone obliterating the oval window

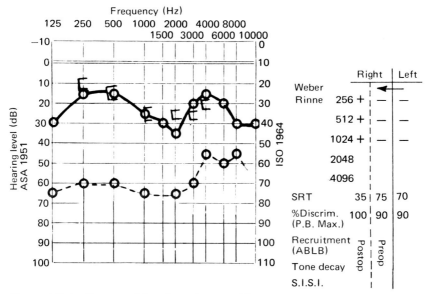

Figure 6.5 Audiogram of female patient aged 35 years, showing hearing gain at 7 years after malleo-vestibulopexy using Teflon piston for case of obliterated footplate. (o—o) Right ear air conduction; ([[) right ear bone conduction; (o---o) right ear air conduction before operation. (From Gristwood and Venables, 1975, courtesy of the Editor and Publishers, *Journal of Laryngology and Otology*)

was hard and 1.5 mm thick. The overlying mucoperiosteum was thin, delicate and avascular.

(15) *Revision surgery* was carried out on 4 cases of delayed conductive hearing loss, but with relatively disappointing results.

RESULTS OF SURGERY

The otologist uses bone conduction measurements to estimate the patient's level of sensorineural reserve, which in turn predicts the postoperative hearing level, since it is the surgeon's hope that the patient will approximate this level after successful stapes surgery. Assuming that the audiometer is in calibration, that the testing environment is acceptable and that the testing technique is both correct and careful, there are several factors which can reduce the accuracy of prediction (Carhart, 1962). These include:

(1) the many variables that differentiate one otosclerotic lesion from another, as well as one operation from the next, and on which the outcome of surgery depends;

(2) the mechanical shift or distortion of bone conduction thresholds (Carhart notch) due to stapes fixation which may itself be atypical, and can vary sufficiently from patient to patient to make use of an average correction of the

Carhart notch significantly inaccurate (no correction for the Carhart notch has been made for our cases);

(3) the limitations of bone conduction audiometry: threshold measurements for some patients with otosclerosis can be in serious error (a) because of false lateralization of the test tone in the absence of adequate masking, (b) hyperdistractibility in the presence of masking noise, and (c) the fact that masking noise becomes ineffective when applied to an ear with substantial hearing impairment. In an attempt to overcome these limitations of the test procedure, the wide-band white noise formerly used for masking in bone conduction tests was replaced in 1966 by the more efficient narrow-band noise delivered by an insert receiver instead of a headphone, thereby increasing the interaural attenuation of the noise and reducing the likelihood of overmasking (Owens, 1972).

There are many and varied methods of analyzing the results of hearing improvement surgery (Tos, 1972) so as to give a clear and comprehensive perspective. Bar diagrams of each patient individually represented are somewhat unwieldy for a large series of cases. *Figure 6.6* shows the results for 49 patients with preoperative bone conduction thresholds of less than 40 dB ISO over the speech frequencies 0.5–2 kHz, and for 41 patients with measurable preoperative bone conduction thresholds between 40 and 70 dB ISO.

Analysis of the data in the large using standard statistical techniques is concerned with several basic questions which include estimating the mean postoperative bone/air gap achieved at various re-examination times and testing for changes with time, as well as studying the influence of other variables particular to the patient.

By the term 'bone/air gap' we mean the difference (in decibels) between the air conduction reading and the preoperative bone conduction reading over the speech frequencies 0.5–2 kHz. *Table 6.2* shows the sample means, standard deviations and the 95% confidence intervals for the mean bone/air gap at each re-examination time considered separately over a period of 10 years.

Table 6.2 Sample means, standard deviations and confidence intervals for mean bone/air (B/A) gap

Examination time	Number	Mean B/A gap	Standard deviation	95% Confidence interval for mean
Preoperatively	140	39.8	9.5	38.2 to 41.3
3 Months	140	4.1	14.1	1.8 to 6.5
1 Year	133	4.4	15.1	1.8 to 7.0
3 Years	122	2.7	14.8	−0.01 to 5.3
5 Years	114	2.1	14.1	−0.5 to 4.7
7 Years	94	5.7	15.8	2.4 to 8.9
10 Years	61/125*	5.3	15.3	1.4 to 9.2

* Fifteen cases not included as their potential follow-up of 10 years had not been reached when the analysis was performed.

A previous study (Gristwood and Venables, 1975) of 100 piston cases confirmed that there was no change of the mean bone/air gap with time (over five years) and that there were no grounds for excluding patients from operation on account of age or the finding of active otosclerosis (soft bone and thickened vascular mucoperiosteum).

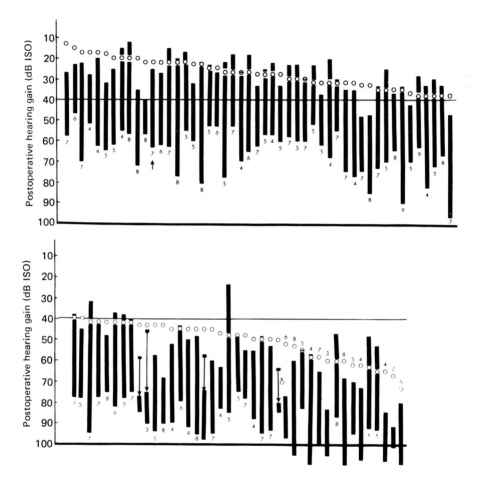

Figure 6.6 The bar diagrams show the postoperative gains of hearing of 90 consecutive cases of obliterative otosclerosis, 49 with bone conduction (BC) levels of less than 40 dB (top) and 41 with BC of more than 40 dB (bottom), arranged in order of decreasing sensorineural function. All cases had a Teflon or wire Teflon piston technique. The open circles represent the preoperative mean bone conduction level over the three frequencies 500, 1000 and 2000 Hz. The vertical height of the black column indicates the gain of hearing for each case at an epoch after surgery denoted in years by the digit appended below (or above) each column. The upper end of the bar is the average air conduction level over 500, 1000 and 2000 Hz at the time of latest assessment. The lower end of each column is the preoperative air conduction reading. A downward pointing arrow (↓) indicates a case with initial hearing improvement that later deteriorated. (From Gristwood and Venables, 1975, courtesy of the Editor and Publishers, *Journal of Laryngology and Otology*)

CONCLUSION

Stapes surgery using some type of solid piston-shaped prosthesis is highly recommended as a suitable and safe method for the long-term alleviation of conductive hearing impairment in patients with obliterative otosclerosis of the oval window, regardless of whether the otosclerosis is active or not.

Acknowledgement

The author acknowledges his indebtedness to Dr William N. Venables of the Department of Statistics, University of Adelaide, for advice and assistance on statistical matters.

References

Bellucci, R. J. (1978) Footplate extraction in stapedectomy. *Laryngoscope*, **88,** 701–706

Carhart, R. (1962) Effect of stapes fixation on bone conduction response. In *Otosclerosis* (Henry Ford Hospital International Symposium), edited by H. F. Schuknecht, pp. 175–197. Boston: Little, Brown and Company

Cody, D. T., Hallberg, O. E. and Simonton, K. M. (1967) Stapedectomy for otosclerosis. Some causes of failure. *Archives of Otolaryngology*, **85,** 184–191

Ford, C. N., Jr, Nichols, R. C., Graham, A. B. and Hayden, R. (1971) Long-term hearing results in obliterative otosclerosis. *Transactions of the American Academy of Ophthalmology and Otology*, **75,** 24–30

Gristwood, R. E. (1966a) Obliterative otosclerosis: an analysis of the clinical and audiometric findings. *Journal of Laryngology and Otology*, **80,** 1115–1126

Gristwood, R. E. (1966b) Obliterative otosclerosis. *Journal of the Oto-Laryngological Society of Australia* 2(1), 40–48

Gristwood, R. E. (1969) Haemostatic injection for otological surgery. *Journal of the Oto-Laryngological Society of Australia*, **2**(4), 39–41

Gristwood, R. E. (1970) The longer-term results of surgery in obliterative otosclerosis. *Journal of the Oto-Laryngological Society of Australia*, 3(1), 61–65

Gristwood, R. E. and Venables, W. N. (1975) Otosclerotic obliteration of the oval window niche: an analysis of the results of surgery. *Journal of Laryngology and Otology*, **89,** 1185–1217

Gristwood, R. E. and Venables, W. N. (1982) A note on progression of the otosclerotic focus. *Clinical Otolaryngology* (in press)

Guilford, F. (1963) Panel on footplate pathology, techniques and prognosis. *Archives of Otolaryngology*, **78,** 520–538

Hall, I. S. (1963) Discussion: stapes surgery for otosclerosis. *Journal of Laryngology and Otology*, **77,** 844

Hall, I. S. and Millar, A. Mc. (1950) Haemostasis in the fenestration operation. *Journal of Laryngology and Otology*, **64,** 233–238

Hough, J. V. D. (1963) Panel on footplate pathology, techniques and prognosis. *Archives of Otolaryngology*, **78,** 520–538

House, H. P. (1962) Footplate surgery in otosclerosis. *Journal of Laryngology and Otology*, **76**, 73–86

Katz, R. L. and Katz, G. J. (1966) Surgical infiltration of pressor drugs and their interaction with volatile anaesthetics. *British Journal of Anaesthesia*, **38**, 712–718

McGee, T. M. (1965) The stainless steel piston. Surgical indications and results. *Archives of Otolaryngology (Chicago)*, **81**, 34–40

Morrison, A. (1979) Otosclerosis. In Scott-Brown's *Diseases of the Ear, Nose and Throat*, 4th Edn., edited by J. Ballantyne and J. Groves, Vol. 2, pp. 405–464. London: Butterworths

Owens, E. (1972) In *Guidelines for Clinical Auditory Evaluation*. Rochester, Minnesota: American Academy of Ophthalmology and Otolaryngology

Plester, D. (1970) Fortschritte in der Mikrochirurgie des Ohres in den letzten 10 Jahren. *HNO (Berlin)*, **18**, 33–40

Plester, D. (1971) Congenital malformation of the middle ear. *Acta Otorhino-laryngologica Belgica (Brussels)*, **25**, 877–884

Schuknecht, H. (1963) Discussion of paper by J. J. Shea. *Transactions of the American Otological Society*, **51**, 181

Schuknecht, H. (1971) *Stapedectomy*, p. 16. Boston: Little, Brown and Company

Shea, J. J., Jr. (1963a) The Teflon piston operation for otosclerosis. *Laryngoscope*, **73**, 508–509

Shea, J. J., Jr. (1963b) Complications of the stapedectomy operation. *Transactions of the American Otological Society*, **51**, 181–200

Shea, J. J., Jr. (1969) A technique for stapes surgery in obliterative otosclerosis. *Otolaryngologic Clinics of North America*, 199–213

Shea, J. J., Sanabria, F. and Smyth, G. D. (1962) Teflon piston operation for otosclerosis. *Archives of Otolaryngology (Chicago)*, **76**, 516–521

Sheehy, J. L. (1964) Far-advanced otosclerosis: diagnostic criteria and results of treatment: report of 67 cases. *Archives of Otolaryngology (Chicago)*, **80**, 244–249

Sleigh, J. D. (1974) Antibiotics and chemotherapeutic agents. In *Scientific Foundations of Surgery*, 2nd Edn., edited by C. Wells, J. Kyle and J. E. Dunphy, pp. 789–795. London: William Heinemann Medical Books Ltd

Sooy, F. A., Owens, E. and Theurer, D. (1964a) Stapedectomy in obliterative otosclerosis. *Annals of Otology, Rhinology and Laryngology (St Louis)*, **73**, 679–694

Sooy, F. A., Owens, E. and Theurer, D. (1964b) Stapedectomy in obliterative otosclerosis. *Transactions of the American Otological Society*, **52**, 59–80

Sullivan, J. A. (1963) Stapes surgery for otosclerosis. *Journal of Laryngology and Otology*, **77**, 840–842

Tos, M. (1972) Assessment of the results of tympanoplasty. *Journal of Laryngology and Otology*, **86**, 487–500

Walsh, T. E. (1965) Fenestration in stapedectomy era. *Archives of Otolaryngology (Chicago)*, **82**, 346–354

Willis, R. C. (1964) Obliterative otosclerosis: an analysis of the surgical results. *Journal of the Oto-Laryngological Society of Australia*, **1**, 294–298

Part 2

Facial nerve and inner ear problems

7
Pathophysiology of facial nerve injury
Roger L. Crumley

INTRODUCTION

In order to understand the diagnostic tests of facial nerve function the clinician needs a basic knowledge of neurophysiology. Likewise, predictions of results from facial nerve surgery are only possible if the surgeon is thoroughly familiar with the neuronal effects of peripheral nerve injuries.

The effects of injuries to the peripheral facial nerve are more extensive than previously believed, and include metabolic and anatomical changes in the brain stem and in the facial muscles. In addition there are probably secondary synaptic changes in the facial nucleus.

This chapter concerns itself with injuries which produce facial paralysis. The normal anatomy and physiology of the peripheral facial nerve, consisting of facial motor neurons in the nucleus and their peripheral fibers as far as the motor end plate, will be reviewed first so that the implications of injury can be more easily understood.

THE PERIPHERAL FACIAL NERVE

Normal anatomy

The facial nerve motor nucleus in the pons is the source of 7000 motor axons which innervate the facial muscles (Fisch and Esslen, 1977). Approximately 3000 other fibers join these motor fibers to make up the entire facial nerve peripheral axon population. These latter fibers are composed of:

(1) special visceral afferent fibers to the taste buds of the anterior two-thirds of the tongue. These fibers have their unipolar cell bodies located in the geniculate ganglion, with central synapses in the nucleus of tractus solitarius;

(2) general visceral efferent secretomotor fibers to the submandibular and sub-lingual salivary glands, the lacrimal gland, and mucous glands of the nose and sinuses. These fibers are derived from the superior salivatory nuclei (Diamond and Frew, 1979);
(3) general somatic afferent fibers which are sensory to the skin of the posterior aspect of the external auditory canal and the concha of the external ear. These fibers have cell bodies located in the Gasserian (trigeminal) ganglion.

Responses to injury of these three types of fibers (in contrast to the motor fibers of the facial nerve) are not entirely understood. Some investigators feel that secretomotor fibers are more sensitive to pressure lesions and take longer to return to normal function. These fibers tend to be smaller in diameter and less myelinated than the large type A motor fibers emanating from the facial motor nucleus (Waxman, 1980).

The motor facial nucleus lies in the lower third of the pons, deep in the reticular formation. The cells are arranged in small groups to form subnuclei, each of which seems to be responsible for innervating the particular muscle supplied by an individual nerve branch, e.g. the rostral subnuclei are concerned with innervation of the frontalis and orbicularis oculi, while caudal subnuclei innervate lower face and platysma muscles. The most rostral subnuclei (forehead and upper portion of orbicularis oculi) receive fibers from both cerebral hemispheres, and therefore have crossed and uncrossed supranuclear innervation (Diamond and Frew, 1979).

Normal function

Each facial nerve neuron is composed of a cell body (soma, perikaryon), several dendrites which receive afferent input from higher centers in the brain, and one peripheral axon. The sheath of each axon consists of a myelin layer internally, a covering layer of Schwann cell cytoplasm, and a connective tissue layer, the endoneurium, externally (*Figure 7.1*). A membrane potential of 90 mV exists across the axon membrane. The total cross-sectional diameter of these fibers ranges from 2 to 30 μm. The sheath is deficient or absent at nodes of Ranvier, which are spaced from 0.1 mm to 1.8 mm apart.

The cell body exchanges biological materials with the entire peripheral component of the neuron. The centrifugal system consists of production of acetylcholine, choline-acetyl transferase, and other substances in the cell body. These substances undergo proximodistal (centrifugal) transport toward the motor end plate (Ducker and Kauffman, 1977). There are at least two different rates of proximodistal axoplasmic flow, the more rapid of which is 17 mm per hour, or approximately 41 cm per day. While most of the peripheral axon and motor end plate nutrition comes from the cell body via this system, some of the distal portion of each fiber is dependent upon local blood vessels for nutrition. For this reason brain stem (nuclear) insults and/or local ischemic lesions can impair peripheral nerve function or nerve regeneration.

Metabolic breakdown of neurotransmitters occurs at the motor end plate. Some of the breakdown products are thought to be carried back to the cell body via distoproximal (centripetal) axoplasmic flow. These flow rates appear to be slower than those associated with proximodistal transport.

When a parent neuron fires in the normal facial nucleus, the facial nerve axon undergoes depolarization, transmitting the impulse distally to the facial muscle fibers. Due to the myelination of the nerve fiber, the wave of depolarization jumps from one node of Ranvier to the next, a process termed 'saltatory conduction'. This

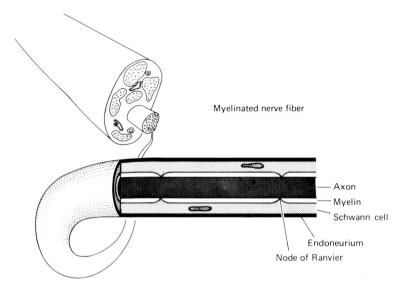

Figure 7.1 Single myelinated axon. Note myelin, Schwann cell and endoneurial layers. These three layers comprise the endoneurial tube

explains the characteristic rapid conduction velocity of the facial nerve, 70 to 100 m/s. After imperfect regeneration of the myelin sheath following injury, or in certain demyelinating lesions, conduction velocity is slowed markedly.

A second function of the myelin sheath appears to be that of providing electrical insulation between adjacent axons. Hence, when this myelin sheath is lost, 'cross-talk' can occur between neighboring fibers. Thus, the depolarization potential of one fiber may skip to a neighboring fiber, producing secondary depolarization. This phenomenon is called *ephapse* and is thought to be one of the explanations for the spasms and synkinesis following imperfect nerve regeneration.

Blood supply

The blood supply of the facial nerve consists of a continuing anastomotic pattern with origin from three vessels (Miehlke, 1973). The most proximal portion of the facial nerve (meatal and labyrinthine segments) is primarily supplied by the labyrinthine artery, a branch of the anterior inferior cerebellar artery (Anson *et al.*, 1970). This vessel anastomoses near the geniculate ganglion with a branch of the middle meningeal artery which arises from the internal maxillary artery of the external carotid system.

Distally, blood from this vessel communicates with blood from the stylomastoid artery from the posterior auricular vessel of the external carotid system. This latter vessel supplies the mastoid segment of the nerve and anastomoses with the superficial petrosal branch in the region of the tympanic segment. In addition small branches from the internal carotid system, the caroticotympanic arteries, contribute to the blood supply of the tympanic segment.

Injury

The cell body and proximal axon

The normal high level of metabolic activity in these neurons is increased markedly following peripheral nerve injury (axotomy). This is seen histologically as cellular swelling, nuclear eccentricity, nucleolar enlargement, and chromatolysis. These changes are associated with an important change in the intracellular enzymatic machinery. Neurotransmitter synthesis ceases and is replaced by the production of proteosynthetic materials (Ducker and Kauffman, 1977). This process has been likened to that of a peacetime automobile factory converting its machinery to the production of tanks in wartime. Hence, following axotomy, neurotransmitter substances decrease, and proteosynthetic materials, such as glucose-6-phosphate dehydrogenase, ribonucleic acid (RNA), and nicotinamide adenine dinucleotide phosphate (NADPH) undergo marked increases. These enzymatic changes, and the histological change with which they are associated, are known as the 'retrograde reaction'.

The term 'retrograde reaction' describes what happens proximally in the injured *axon*. However, the most important changes occur in the *cell body* and perhaps should be termed instead 'cell body response'. Cell bodies in the nucleus increase in size shortly following axotomy, although the cause for this change in size is not clear. There are significant changes in RNA synthesis which are thought to depend upon some process of gene activation. This increase in ribosomal RNA is thought to presage an increase in protein synthesis. Neurotransmitter production falls sharply following axotomy. This phenomenon cannot be explained by simple 'leakage' from the cut axon tip, since the overall result is a net increase in total protein synthesis. Other changes include proliferation of smooth endoplasmic reticulum, increased lipid synthesis, and certain changes in energy metabolism. Changes in axoplasmic flow are not observed until after the metabolic transformation takes place in the cell body (Grafstein, 1975).

Other nuclear changes

During the time of maximal cellular swelling, there is a loosening of the attachment between the neuron and its neighboring glia. Metabolic changes also occur in the dendrites. A significant retraction of the dendritic field has been observed. Dendritic loss of presynaptic boutons and depletion of transmitter-associated protein have also been described (Kreutzberg, 1973).

The glial and interstitial fluid environment of the cell body is also altered markedly by peripheral nerve injury. Neighboring microglial cells undergo mitoses and proliferation in the first week following nerve injury. These proliferating microglial cells cover most of the surface area of the cell body and its dendrites. This produces displacement of the terminal boutons. These boutons are removed by microglial processes, leaving the neurons with a reduced or absent afferent input. Changes in these supranuclear synapses may very well play an important role in the origin of mass movements, disturbances of fine movements, and affective movements. Loss or imperfect regeneration of inhibitory synapses might produce spasms of the facial nerve, while inappropriate regeneration of the synapses with 'mismatching' would cause frank synkinesis.

In most cases the cell body recovers at about the same time as axon regrowth is complete to the periphery. The final condition of the cell body is influenced by the type of functional reconnection made, e.g. whether the nerve is reconnected to a similar muscle fiber, or inappropriate regeneration occurs to a sensory end organ, glandular element, or other inappropriate distal member. A significant observation, however, is that when reconnection of the regenerating axon is prevented, the decline in proteosynthetic materials occurs *at the same time* as it would have done if neural reconnection had occurred. This suggests that once the cell body reaction is initiated, it runs its course without feedback from the regenerating axon, presumably according to a pre-set genetic program (Grafstein, 1975).

The initiation of cell body response appears to be due to a 'signal compound' which is transported from the injury site proximally to the cell body. It is estimated that such a signal ascends the axon at a rate of several millimeters per day. The time required for the appearance of these changes is proportional to the distance between the cell body and the lesion (Ducker and Kauffman, 1977).

Axon regeneration does not occur immediately following peripheral nerve injury (axotomy). It takes approximately 3 weeks for these changes to reach maximal levels. Some investigators feel that this period represents the optimal time to wait before performing reparative nerve surgery (McCabe, 1977).

Animal research has shown that trimming of the severed nerve ends at 3 weeks produces a secondary increase in axoplasmic transport rates (McQuarrie and Grafstein, 1973). Other investigators, however, notably Sunderland, feel that such trimming of the proximal stump at the injury site necessitates a second 'retrograde reaction', and results in a secondary decrement in axon regeneration rates (Sunderland, 1980).

The amount and rate of axon regeneration appear to be enhanced by administration of thyroid hormone and growth hormone. Distal sprouting of the axon also appears to be enhanced by these substances. To date, however, clinical use of this positive pharmacological action has been limited.

CLASSIFICATION OF INJURY

When the peripheral axon is severed, the muscle, motor end plate, distal fragment of axon, proximal portion, and cell body undergo marked metabolic derangements and transformations. Likewise, the environment surrounding the cell body is grossly altered. The following describes the effects of increasing 'degrees' of injury at the site of lesion in peripheral injuries (Sunderland, 1972).

In the early 1940s, Seddon produced a classification of nerve injuries that was quite useful at the time: neurapraxia, axonotmesis, and neurotmesis. The classic description of these injuries, however, was somewhat difficult to correlate with the clinical situation (Seddon, 1944).

Sunderland's classification ('first degree through fifth degree of injury') makes it possible to understand the effect of injury on each individual axon, and on the nerve trunk itself.

First degree injury (conduction block)

This type of nerve fiber injury is analogous to Seddon's 'neurapraxia' and is also called conduction block injury (*Figure 7.2*). Notice that the axon and its endoneurial tube are slightly indented, twisted or otherwise distorted. The Schwann sheath, myelin layer, endoneurium and axon are all in continuity. Both distoproximal and proximodistal axoplasmic transport continue. The nerve fiber distal to the site of

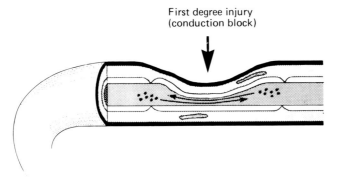

Figure 7.2 First degree injury (conduction block). Note indentation of axon and endoneurial tube (arrow). All structures, including the axon, are in continuity

injury retains *normal* electrical response. Normally propagated waves of depolarization from the cell body, however, and electrical stimulation proximal to the site of lesion, evoke no distal response, since conduction is blocked. As long as axon continuity is preserved and axoplasmic flow continues in both directions, this physiological and electrical situation will persist.

To correlate one axon's first degree injury with the clinical situation requires some extrapolation. If all 7000 motor fibers in one facial nerve are in a first degree of injury, the nerve will remain electrically stimulable. In fact the distal facial nerve should stimulate at the same level of electrical stimulation as the normal opposite side. Since all 7000 endoneurial tubes (Schwann sheath and myelin layer) are intact, the facial function will be fully restored when the block is cleared. Ordinarily there will be no permanent sequelae from such an injury.

Although the above hypothetical situation is helpful in understanding the first degree of injury, only rarely would *all* 7000 of the motor fibers be involved with a first degree injury as described. Almost all nerve injuries are 'mixed'. For example, if 2000 to 3000 fibers were conducting normally while the other 4000 to 5000 fibers were in the first degree of injury, the distal portion of normal fibers *and* fibers in first degree of injury would be similarly capable of electrical stimulation. Likewise, evoked electromyography, also called 'electroneuronography' (ENOG), would 'count' a normal number of intact distal axons. In ENOG, if the stimulator tip could be placed proximal to the site of lesion, normal fibers would conduct the stimulated depolarization wave normally while those in a first degree of injury would 'block' the wave of propagation. This, of course, is the basis for intra-operative ENOG, as described by Fisch and Esslen (1977).

Recovery in first degree injuries is usually quite rapid, most commonly less than 3 weeks, since the cell body does not have to regenerate a peripheral axon.

Second degree injury (loss of axon continuity with preservation of endoneurial tube)

With regard to the amount of injury inflicted on a single axon, second degree injury implies an increasing force of indentation, twisting, or distortion (*Figure 7.3*). Note that in this injury the axon is compressed to the extent that continuity is disrupted. Neurotransmitter substances manufactured in the cell body can no longer reach the

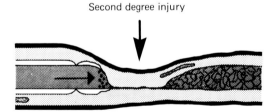

Second degree injury

Figure 7.3 Second degree injury. Axon is discontinuous, resulting in distal Wallerian degeneration. Endoneurial tube structures (particularly Schwann cell and endoneurium) remain intact

motor end plate region, and neural metabolites from the muscle and motor end plate cannot pass proximally to the cell body. This loss of axon continuity makes a second degree injury much more detrimental to the entire neuron than a first degree injury for the following reasons:

(1) A 'biological signal' tells the cell body that the distal axon has been interrupted.
(2) This invokes the 'metabolic transformation' described earlier
(3) The distal axon undergoes Wallerian degeneration
(4) Various biochemical and histological alterations occur in muscle and in the brain stem due to this denervation.

The proximal axon segment now acts as a communication conduit from cell body to site of injury. The proximal segment retains its endoneurial tube structures, as does the distal segment in this degree of injury. This proximal segment is to become (in 14 to 21 days) a conduit for proteosynthetic substances which will allow axon regeneration. (Remember that the distal axon must regenerate to the motor end plate for recovery to occur.)

At the site of lesion the endoneurial tube retains continuity, although there is often some thinning of the myelin layer. The perineurium surrounding the fascicle, and the fascicular arrangement of the nerve, remain intact. Retention of endoneurial tube continuity allows the nerve to regenerate to its former identical muscle fiber(s), and permits normal neuromuscular function, provided that axon regeneration is complete.

Axon regeneration

Axon regeneration is necessary for return of function in second, third, fourth and fifth degree injuries, and consequently will be discussed at this point.

Ordinarily, the axon sprouts do not enter the distal segment for a period of 7 to 21 days. The mechanisms for this regeneration are incompletely understood. It appears that with distal lesions this sprouting may occur somewhat later, although regeneration will be more complete since the neuron has sustained less of an amputation injury. In proximal lesions axon sprouting may occur earlier, provided that the more proximal injury does not result in death of the cell body.

Once axon sprouting and growth begin, the new axons grow at the rate of approximately 1 mm per day. The distance from injury to the motor end plate, nutritional factors, age and type of injury all affect the length of the recovery period and the quality of resultant function. Blunt injuries appear to induce a heightened cell body response, and are more likely to result in neuron death than sharp transections.

Location of the injury appears to be an important factor in determining extent of central changes. Proximal injuries (cerebellopontine angle, meatal portion, labyrinthine portion) cause greater nuclear change because a larger portion of the neuron is amputated. In contrast, a laceration of a small distal facial nerve branch leaves the long axonal process intact, requiring less regeneration for the nerve to return to its motor end plate (Ducker and Kauffman, 1977).

Age is probably the most important factor in nerve regeneration. All experienced surgeons in the field have noted that youth has a most positive influence on neural regeneration. This may be due to the presence of growth hormone in children, as this hormone appears to be similar to nerve growth factor. Clinical trials of such substances in promoting nerve regeneration are inconclusive at this time. There is evidence that thyroid hormone also promotes nerve regeneration; again, clinical trials have not been completed to confirm this hypothesis.

Marked species differences are known to exist with regard to nerve regeneration. Certain lizards will regrow entire segments of spinal cord when their tail has been amputated. Rats and dogs have less regenerative potential, while baboons, chimpanzees, and man are least capable of nerve regeneration.

Certain types of nerve wounds (massive blast injury, war injuries) may result in *devascularization* of the proximal and/or distal peripheral nerve. This kind of wound promotes excessive scar tissue and delays healing, both of which adversely affect subsequent nerve regeneration. Patients with multiple injuries may become *catabolic* for 2 to 3 months and this, too, adversely influences nerve regeneration.

Even after the regenerating axon reaches the periphery, the fiber is not ready to conduct normally until the cell body switches its enzymatic machinery back to those biochemical processes concerned with excitation and conduction. This takes from 60 to 90 days following the completion of axon regeneration.

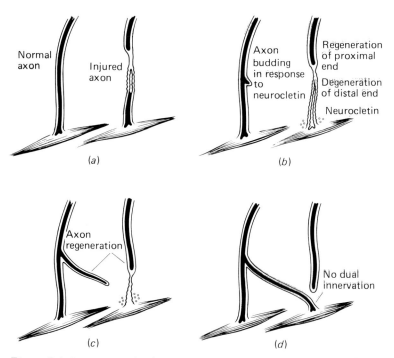

Figure 7.4 Axon sprouting in muscle. The normal axon (on the left) sprouts in response to neurochemical substances ('neurocletin') elaborated by the denervated motor end plate. This precludes reinnervation by the original injured axon (on the right)

It is probable that metabolic factors in the denervated muscle promote axon sprouting. This results in a change in configuration of motor units (a motor unit is defined as the muscle fibers innervated by one motor neuron) and corresponding changes in electromyographic patterns. However, if all 7000 axons are afflicted with second degree injury, and axon regeneration is complete, it is likely that normal EMG patterns will result.

It must be remembered that the above discussion stipulates that all 7000 fibers are found in a state of second degree injury. If on the other hand 2000 fibers were normal, another 2000 in first degree injury, and the remaining 3000 in second degree injury, the regenerative situation is changed. The normal fibers will remain normal. The first degree injury fibers will reinnervate their normal muscle fibers following cessation of the conduction block. The regenerating fibers which are in second degree injury will arrive at the muscle several months following the injury. By this time some of the muscle fibers previously innervated by these axons will have become innervated by intramuscular axon sprouting from the normal and the first degree injury fibers. Thus, although we would expect normal distal regeneration of axons from the second degree injury fibers in this situation, intramuscular factors, including axon sprouting, have allowed the less seriously injured axons to reinnervate muscle fibers previously innervated by axons in second degree injury (*Figure 7.4*).

Third degree injury (disruption of axon and endoneurial tube)

Third degree injury (*Figure 7.5*) results from a greater force of indentation, twisting, or distortion than first or second degree injuries. Note that in this injury the axon *and the endoneurial tube* become discontinuous at the site of lesion.

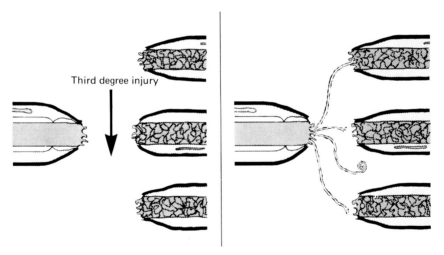

Figure 7.5 Third degree injury. Axon *and* endoneurial tube are disrupted. This results in misdirected regeneration or loss of many regenerating axons

The immediate consequences of this injury are those of Wallerian degeneration, much as with second degree injury. However, during axon regeneration the tiny axon sprouts are free to enter *any* distal endoneurial tube available, curl up in between distal endoneurial tubules, or wander elsewhere within the nerve fascicle. This allows one or more of the following: (1) one axon sprout to enter the correct endoneurial tube; (2) another axon sprout (from the same proximal axon) to enter an 'incorrect' distal tubule; (3) loss of many axon sprouts which fail to enter any tubule (*Figure 7.5*).

If axon regeneration is complete, distal muscle strength may be nearly normal, except that 'mass movements', or synkinesis, will develop because proximal axons no longer pass distally to the same muscles as prior to injury. This is at least one of the possible causes of synkinesis in such lesions. Other possibilities include *ephapse* and central changes, which will be described below (Crumley, 1979b).

Fourth degree injury

Fourth degree injury is defined as disruption of perineurium surrounding nerve fascicles, with preservation of the nerve sheath. In this type of injury, a force is exerted on the nerve sufficient to rupture the fascicular containment layer, the perineurium (*Figure 7.6*). All axons within the fascicle undergo third degree injury, while the fourth degree is added to indicate that a greater force was needed to cause the injury, and that a poorer result will follow nerve regeneration.

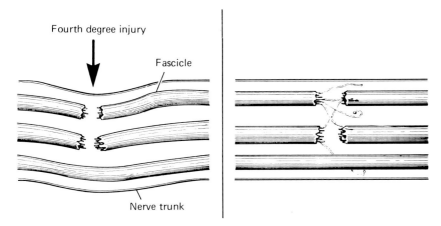

Figure 7.6 Fourth degree injury. Increasing compression or torsion causes disruption of perineurium, allowing axons to regenerate beyond their original fascicle

As perineurium no longer confines regenerating axon sprouts to their appropriate fascicle, they are free to regenerate into the interfascicular sheath and be lost in neuroma formation, or to regenerate into a distal endoneurial tubule within an adjacent fascicle. This will result in a decreased axon population as the regenerating fibers reach the periphery and therefore a 'less concentrated' innervation of the facial muscle. It may well be that the fewer axons reaching the periphery sprout sufficiently to innervate *all* the motor end plates previously innervated, but the insufficient number of axons will usually result in less muscle contraction following this degree of injury.

Fifth degree injury

If the nerve trunk is entirely disrupted the lesion is termed fifth degree or, in the older terminology, neurotmesis. This means that, in addition to disruption of the axon, endoneurium and perineurium, the sheath surrounding the nerve has been

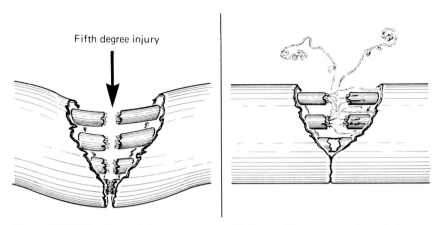

Figure 7.7 Fifth degree injury (neurotmesis). In addition to axon loss during regeneration (as described for the second, third, and fourth degrees of injury), extraneural regeneration occurs in this injury

torn. Again, all axons of the nerve will undergo Wallerian degeneration and subsequently mount a regenerative effort. However, in this injury axon sprouts are not only free to regenerate to the periphery, as with the other degrees, but also have the potential to regenerate outside the nerve and be lost in extraneural gliomata (*Figure 7.7*). This is the type of injury seen with all sharp complete transections. Naturally, these injuries result in synkinesis and muscle weakness.

DEGREES OF INJURY AND NERVE EXCITABILITY TESTING

If nerve injuries were always purely first or second degree, the results of nerve excitability testing would be easy to interpret. Naturally, if all 7000 fibers had undergone a first degree injury, electrical excitability (stimulability) on the face would be normal. If all 7000 fibers had sustained a second degree injury, electrical excitability would disappear between 48 and 96 hours. This would also be true for third, fourth, and fifth degree injuries.

However, clinicians are not frequently given the luxury of such pure diseases or injuries. Most injuries to the facial nerve contain a mixture of the various degrees. The effects of these mixed lesions on excitability testing are not yet known. However, since excitability testing is *normal* with all fibers in a first degree of injury and *absent* if all fibers are in a second degree of injury, most patients who have intermediate results with nerve excitability testing most probably have mixed lesions. For example, a patient with a temporal bone fracture and increasing edema at the fracture site might have 1000 normal axons, 3000 with first degree injury, and the other 3000 with second degree injury and beyond. As 4000 fibers would still be 'in continuity', the nerve excitability test might show an elevated threshold, perhaps 5 or 6 mA.

On the other hand, if no fibers were normal, 2000 fibers were in first degree injury, and the remaining 5000 in second and third degrees of injury, the nerve might show absent or nearly absent nerve excitability. (It is not known how many fibers are necessary to conduct electrical excitation to the periphery.) This is the type of lesion which may allow so-called 'immediate return of function' following facial nerve decompression (McCabe, 1977). This could hypothetically result from releasing the conduction block of the 2000 fibers in first degree of injury and allowing them to resume normal function.

All this is highly speculative, and more research is needed in this area and with nerve excitability testing. Evoked electromyography (electroneuronography) may one day be able to 'count' the number of fibers which are normal and those which are in first degree injury in these mixed lesions. At present, however, we remain unable to predict the fiber breakdown of such mixed lesions.

THE MOTOR END PLATE REGION

Facial nerve axons normally innervate a number of muscle fibers which is intermediate between the huge motor units of the extremity muscles (2000 muscle fibers per axon in sartorius) and those of the extraocular muscles or laryngeal muscles (2 to 10 muscle fibers per axon). When a peripheral axon undergoes transection, all its motor end plates change their biochemical composition. These changes are somewhat similar to those described in the nerve cell body in the brain stem. An increase in muscle ribonucleic acid, ribosomes, and rough endoplasmic reticulum is seen in the early denervation period. This is presumably to allow proteosynthesis, which may become necessary because of the breakdown of contractile proteins in the muscle cell. It has also been suggested that the new ribosomes may be synthesizing a protein receptor substance for acetylcholine, since it is well known that acetylcholine sensitivity spreads to cover the entire muscle fiber following denervation, rather than being concentrated solely at the motor end plate zone (Sanes, Marshall and McMahon, 1980).

Certain substances elaborated from the motor end plate region are known to induce axon sprouting following denervation. Neurocletin and a substance similar to nerve growth factor have been described as promoting axon sprouting in this region (Hoffman, 1950). It is known that these substances will promote axon sprouting from a normal distal nerve fiber towards a denervated muscle fiber (Diamond *et al.*, 1976). An 'axon sprouting inhibitor factor' has also been described. This biochemical substance, normally found near the motor end plate, prevents axon sprouting in the intact neuromuscular unit. Following axotomy, the absence of this factor is thought to allow axon sprouting, as does the active elaboration of the two substances described above.

If no neural regeneration occurs, the muscle fiber may (1) be reinnervated by adjacent muscles and/or nerves via axon sprouting; (2) remain quiescent in a denervated state for a period of time, expectantly awaiting the arrival of reinnervating axons; (3) undergo atrophy (following a period of time), and eventually even disappear and be replaced by fibrous tissue.

The length of time from denervation to atrophy is highly controversial. Basic investigations have concluded that the time before severe atrophy occurs may be as short as 2 to 3 years. However, clinical observers have performed successful reinnervation surgery as late as 15 to 20 years following paralysis, indicating that the denervated muscle was preserved. The reason for this discrepancy is most probably that neural regeneration following severe nerve injuries is inadequate to induce actual muscle contraction, yet via axon sprouting is capable of occupying the motor end plates and transporting the necessary supply of neurometabolites to the motor end plate region from the cell bodies in the facial nucleus. In that instance, the muscle fibers would be 'preserved' until a reinnervation procedure or resolution of the proximal nerve injury allowed axons to regenerate into the muscle. An extremely important aspect of this phenomenon is that innervated muscle fibers, even though innervated by axons too 'diluted' to produce movement, will not accept new innervation. Hence it is probably important to transect this pre-existing innervation prior to introducing a neural reinnervation source.

CENTRAL PHENOMENA

The effects of peripheral injury on the facial nucleus and supranuclear afferent systems are only partially understood. Kreutzberg (1973) has described increased mitotic activity of perineuronal cells following facial nerve axotomy. Microglial processes from such cells appear to cover the surfaces and synaptic terminals of such facial nerve cell bodies. It is not clear what the end result of these nuclear changes might be, but it is possible that synaptic 'mismatching' occurs following restoration of the cell body to neural transmission (Kreutzberg, 1973).

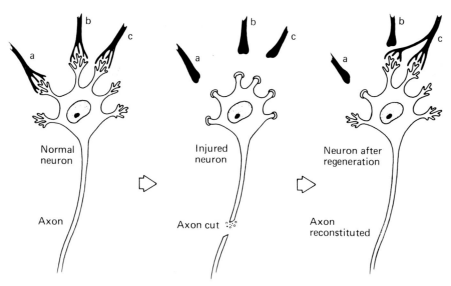

Figure 7.8 Facial nerve cell body in normal (*left*), injured (*center*), and regenerated (*right*) states (artist's conception). Note that after regeneration, one supranuclear fiber (*c*) synapses with two different dendrites, while synaptic connection of another supranuclear fiber (*b*) is blocked

It is well known that the facial nucleus has multiple supranuclear afferent systems acting upon it. Voluntary facial movements ('show your teeth'; 'wrinkle your forehead') originate in the precentral gyrus of the cerebral cortex. These cortico-bulbar fibers pass downward through the posterior part of the internal capsule and most then cross the caudal pons to synapse in the opposite facial nucleus.

Emotional (involuntary) movements, such as smiling, laughing, or eye blinking, are mediated by the hypothalamus, globus pallidus, interneurons in the reticular formation, and brain stem reflex arcs. This explains how the patient with a cerebral vascular accident and infarction of the internal capsule may smile spontaneously when amused, yet be unable to voluntarily 'show his teeth'. Conversely, patients with postencephalitic Parkinsonism (lesions of the globus pallidus) frequently can voluntarily move their faces normally but show no emotional involuntary movements. Other supranuclear afferents affecting the facial nucleus include those from the superior colliculus of the optic system (blink reflex), the superior olive of the auditory system (stapedius reflex), sensory trigeminal nucleus (corneal reflex), and the nucleus of tractus solitarius (chewing and sucking following introduction of food into the mouth) (Crumley, 1979a).

Since it is presumed that each facial nerve cell body derives input from several if not all of these sources, mismatching of these supranuclear inputs might well result in spasms and synkinesis seen following peripheral nerve injuries (*Figure 7.8*). This provides yet another possible explanation for synkinetic movements following peripheral nerve injuries.

SUMMARY

The purpose of this chapter is to acquaint the surgeon with the changes in facial nerve neurons that occur following facial nerve injury. Processes in the peripheral nerve, the muscle, the facial nucleus, and even the supranuclear brain stem have been described and discussed. It is hoped that this will result in improved understanding of these nerve injuries and a more physiological approach to their treatment.

References

Anson, B. J., Donaldson, J. A., Warpeha, R. L. and Rensink, M. J. (1970) The facial nerve, sheath, and blood supply in relation to the surgery of decompression. *Annals of Otology, Rhinology and Laryngology*, **79**, 710–727

Crumley, R. (1979a) The opercular syndrome – diagnostic trap in facial paralysis. *Laryngoscope*, **89**, 361–365

Crumley, R. (1979b) Mechanisms of synkinesis. *Laryngoscope*, **89**, 1847–1854

Diamond, J., Cooper, E., Turner, C. and MacIntyre, L. (1976) Trophic regulation of nerve sprouting. *Science*, **193**, 371–377

Diamond, C. and Frew, I. (1979) *The Facial Nerve*, p. 12. New York and London: Oxford University Press

Ducker, T. B. and Kauffman, F. (1977) Metabolic factors in surgery of peripheral nerves (Proceedings of 1976 Congress of Neurological Surgeons). *Clinical Neurosurgery*, **24**, 406–412

Fisch, U. and Esslen, E. (1977) In *The Acute Facial Palsies*, edited by E. Esslen, pp. 45–49. Heidelberg: Springer-Verlag

Grafstein, B. (1975) The nerve cell body response to axotomy. *Experimental Neurology*, **48** (Part 2), 32–51

Hoffman, H. (1950) Local reinnervation in partially denervated muscle; a histopathological study. *Australian Journal of Experimental Biology and Medical Science*, **28**, 383–397

Kreutzberg, G. W. (1973) *Surgery of the Facial Nerve*, edited by A. Miehlke, pp. 22–29. Philadelphia: W. B. Saunders

McCabe, B. (1977) Some evidence for the efficacy of decompression for Bell's palsy: immediate motion postoperatively. *Laryngoscope*, **87**, 246–249

McQuarrie, I. G. and Grafstein, B. (1973) Axon outgrowth enhanced by a previous nerve injury. *Archives of Neurology*, **29**, 53–55

Miehlke, A. (1973) *Surgery of the Facial Nerve*, 1st Edn, pp. 20–21. Philadelphia: W. B. Saunders

Sanes, T., Marshall, L. and McMahon, U. (1980) Reinnervation of muscle. In *Nerve Repair and Regeneration*, edited by D. L. Jewett and H. R. McCarroll, pp. 130–141. St Louis: C. V. Mosby

Seddon, H. J. (1944) Early management of peripheral nerve injuries. *Practitioner*, **152**, 101–110

Sunderland, S. (1972) *Nerves and Nerve Injuries*, pp. 129–137. London: Churchill Livingstone

Sunderland, S. (1980) Clinical and experimental approaches to nerve repair. In *Nerve Repair and Regeneration*, edited by D. L. Jewett and H. R. McCarroll, pp. 343–344. St Louis: C. V. Mosby

Waxman, S. (1980) Structure-function relations in nerves and nerve injuries. In *Nerve Repair and Regeneration*, edited by D. L. Jewett and H. R. McCarroll, pp. 186–197. St Louis: C. V. Mosby

8
Recent advances in cochlear physiology

E. F. Evans

INTRODUCTION

Over the past 20 years in particular, the cochlea has received an enormous amount of attention from the physiologist. The two main reasons for this attention form the focus of this brief review, and are of relevance to our understanding of sensori-neural hearing loss of cochlear origin.

First has been the demonstration that the cochlea is more than merely a particularly sensitive microphone. It carries out the substantial part of a most important function of the auditory system, namely frequency analysis, i.e. the ability to resolve or filter complex sounds like speech into their component frequencies. On this depends much of our ability to hear speech sounds clearly, especially in competing noise. While we do not fully understand how this remarkable filtering action of the cochlea is brought about, we know that it requires energy and is physiologically vulnerable. Consequently it is easily impaired in pathological conditions of the cochlea.

This leads to the second reason for the contemporary interest in the cochlea. Experimental models of pathological conditions of the cochlea can be readily set up in animals, and have helped to account for a number of features of cochlear hearing loss in physiological terms, particularly recruitment and deterioration in speech intelligibility. As a result of these studies new tools for diagnosis and new aids for rehabilitation are beginning to emerge.

Finally, very recent physiological studies of the effects of various agents on the animal cochlea appear to offer a potential animal model of tinnitus.

FREQUENCY ANALYSIS BY THE COCHLEA

In everyday use the ear has to analyze complex sounds like speech. These contain two or more frequency components which have to be separated for the speech sounds to be recognized. This process of separating simultaneously occurring frequency components from one another is called frequency analysis, frequency resolution or frequency selectivity. This is a most important function of the ear, and yet rather neglected compared to the better known function of frequency discrimination. This is the ability of the ear to discriminate one frequency from another when presented sequentially, not simultaneously. The two functions, frequency selectivity and frequency discrimination, may well be related (Evans, 1978a), but for the purposes of understanding speech, the former is the more important.

It has long been known that, within certain limits, the ear is capable of remarkably good frequency analysis, but it has been an open question as to where this frequency analysis takes place. Recent physiological and psychophysical evidence now suggests that this most important function is largely accomplished at the level of the cochlea. In the cochlea, the peripheral auditory system is supplied

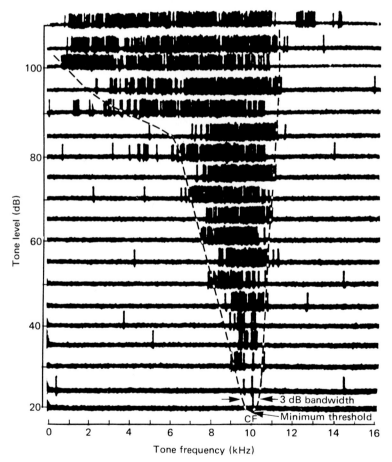

Figure 8.1a Microelectrode record from a single fibre in the cochlear nerve of a guinea-pig showing response to a continuous tone swept in frequency in 5 dB steps of successively higher signal levels. Alternate sweeps are in opposite direction. Spikes are monophasically positive and 0.9 mV in amplitude. Sweep rate linear: 14 kHz/s. The outline (– – –) of the frequency response area thus defined is the frequency threshold curve (FTC). The characteristic frequency (CF) is 10 kHz (*see text*)

with a bank of remarkably sharply tuned filters, each of which filter out of a complex sound, signals within a relatively narrow bandwidth of frequency (*for reviews see* Evans, 1975a, 1978a, 1981).

The cochlea's filtering ability is best understood by reference to the properties of the afferent nerve fibres passing from the cochlea to the central auditory nervous system, in the cochlear or auditory nerve. *Figure 8.1a* shows the result, from a single cochlear nerve fibre, of sweeping a pure tone up and down in frequency at increasing sound levels across the cochlear fibre's frequency response area. The spike responses are the individual action potentials of that cochlear nerve fibre recorded by a microelectrode inserted into it. Outside the cochlear fibre's frequency response area only occasional action potential spikes occur

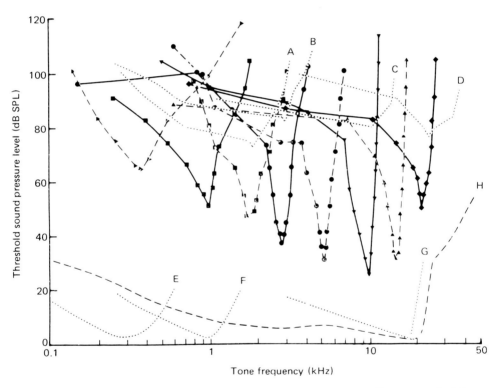

Tone frequency (kHz)

Figure 8.1b Frequency threshold curves (FTCs) of single cochlear fibres recorded from normal and abnormal cochleas (*top*), compared with analogous data for the basilar membrane (*bottom*) of the guinea pig. The continuous and dashed lines through the data points represent FTCs of eight cochlear fibres from six normal cochleas. (Curves A to C) FTCs of cochlear fibres from cochleas rendered abnormal by circulatory inadequacy (CFs at 1.9, 3 and 10 kHz). (D) The curve of highest CF (24 kHz) was obtained in an otherwise normal cochlea (*see text*). (*Bottom*) Analogous curves derived from the measurements of the vibration amplitude of the guinea-pig basilar membrane, by von Békésy (1944: curves E and F); by Johnstone, Taylor and Boyle (1970: curve G) and by Wilson and Johnstone (1975: curve H). All threshold curves are corrected to sound pressure level (in dB SPL) at the tympanic membrane under closed bulla conditions. The basilar membrane curves are positioned arbitrarily on the ordinate scale. (Modified from Evans, 1972)

spontaneously. Within the frequency response area, however, the cochlear fibre responds by generating a continuous burst of spikes. This is its excitatory response, the only response given by cochlear fibres to single tones. The outline of the roughly triangular response area is known as the frequency threshold or 'tuning' curve (FTC). *Figure 8.1b* shows a family of such FTCs plotted for 8 cochlear nerve fibres, each originating from a different position along the cochlear partition. The curve centred at 10 kHz is in fact the frequency threshold curve shown in *Figure 8.1a*. The frequency corresponding to the tip of each FTC is called the characteristic frequency (CF) of that fibre. It is the frequency at which the fibre's response is most sensitive. The characteristic frequency of a cochlear fibre therefore obviously depends on the position along the cochlear partition from which it originates: curves with lower CFs are of cochlear fibres taking origin from the apical low-frequency end of the cochlea, and those with higher CFs from the high-frequency basal end.

The cochlear fibre frequency thresholds represent quite formidable filters. An engineer would measure the FTC bandwidth 3 dB up from the tip (the half power bandwidth) and would find it to be one third to one sixth of an octave wide. The cut-off slopes from the tip of the FTC to the 'skirts' are very steep, exceeding several hundred dB per octave, particularly on the high-frequency side and for cochlear fibres with CFs above about 2 kHz. A characteristic of these cochlear fibres is that the steep low-frequency cut-off becomes suddenly less steep to form a 'low-frequency tail' at about 70 to 90 dB SPL. Cochlear fibres with CFs below 2 kHz have more symmetrical FTCs, and the cut-off slopes become progressively less steep as the CF decreases.

Any auditory stimulus having energy that falls within the FTC of a cochlear fibre will, in principle, evoke an excitatory response from it. Furthermore, the temporal pattern of discharge of cochlear nerve fibres with CFs up to about 3 to 4 kHz will be dominated by the frequencies at the tip of the FTC. This means that, for complex signals like speech, the response of each individual cochlear nerve fibre will be governed, both in terms of the number of discharges per second (the mean discharge rate) and the temporal pattern of the discharges (for low CF cochlear fibres), by the frequency components falling within their frequency response area. These generalizations, however, apply strictly only at lower intensities.

At higher intensities, certain non-linearities make themselves felt. The two most important of these are saturation and lateral suppression. As the level of a stimulus is increased above threshold, a cochlear fibre produces a progressively greater rate of spike discharges over a dynamic range of, on average, 40 dB. Thereafter its discharge rate saturates, and further increases in stimulus level are ineffective in increasing the rate further (*see Figure 8.9b*). The second type of non-linearity concerns the interaction between two or more stimuli of differing frequency, the so-called 'two-tone inhibition' (Sachs and Kiang, 1968), better termed 'lateral suppression'. This does not appear to be a neurally mediated phenomenon, but some sort of non-linear interaction, possibly of a mechanical nature, in the basilar membrane–organ of Corti complex. The effect is that the response to a signal at a fibre's CF can be reduced or suppressed by a signal of higher level, particularly at lower frequencies. Likewise, the temporal discharge pattern of low CF fibres can be dominated by lower frequency signals at high stimulus levels (Rose *et al.*, 1974; Young and Sachs, 1979; *for review see* Evans, 1975a).

These filtering characteristics of the cochlear nerve fibres are important for our understanding of how the ear analyzes complex sounds because, to a first approximation, they can account for the known psychoacoustic frequency selectivity of the ear (*Figure 8.2*). One of the oldest psychoacoustic measurements of the ear's filtering ability is the so-called 'critical band'. This is the bandwidth within which auditory signals are known to sum and interact, and outside which frequencies can be 'heard out' as separate. An analogous measure of the frequency selectivity of cochlear nerve fibres is their effective bandwidth (Evans and Wilson, 1973). This is approximately the bandwidth 3 dB up from the tip (the half power bandwidth). These values are shown in *Figure 8.2* for five cats, and compared with the critical band in man. The effective bandwidths of the cochlear nerve fibres in

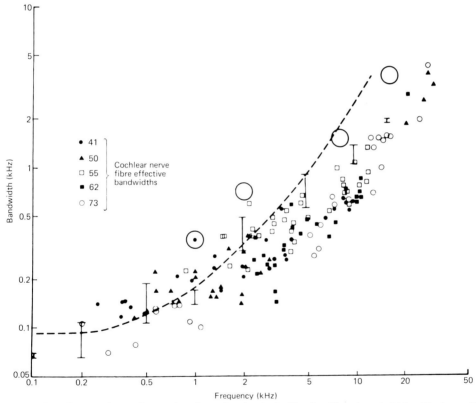

Figure 8.2 Comparison of neural and psychophysical effective filter bandwidths. Each small symbol represents the effective bandwidth of an individual cochlear nerve fibre filter plotted against its characteristic frequency. Individual cats are identified by different symbols. The interrupted line represents the 'critical band' of human hearing, one estimate of the bandwidth of human auditory filters determined psychophysically. The vertical lines represent human effective bandwidths determined by comb-filtered noise masking. Large open circles: behavioural measurements of 'critical band' in the cat. (Modified from Evans and Wilson, 1973; Pickles, 1975)

cats approximate to the values of the human critical bands at the lower frequencies, becoming smaller than the latter for frequencies above about 1 kHz (Evans and Wilson, 1973). Recently, direct measurements of the psychoacoustic critical band have been made in the cat itself (Pickles, 1975). These are indicated in *Figure 8.2* by

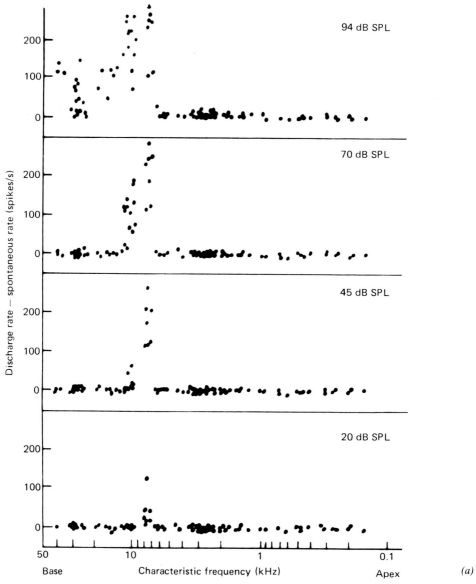

Figure 8.3 Distribution of evoked activity across cat cochlear nerve fibre array in response to single frequencies at different sound levels. Each point represents the increase in discharge rate above spontaneous activity for a given single cochlear nerve fibre plotted at its characteristic frequency (and therefore inferred position along the cochlear partition). (*a*) Responses to 8 kHz tone at four sound levels. (Modified from Evans, 1981) (*b*) Responses to 1 kHz tone at three sound levels. (Modified from Kim and Molnar, 1979.)

111

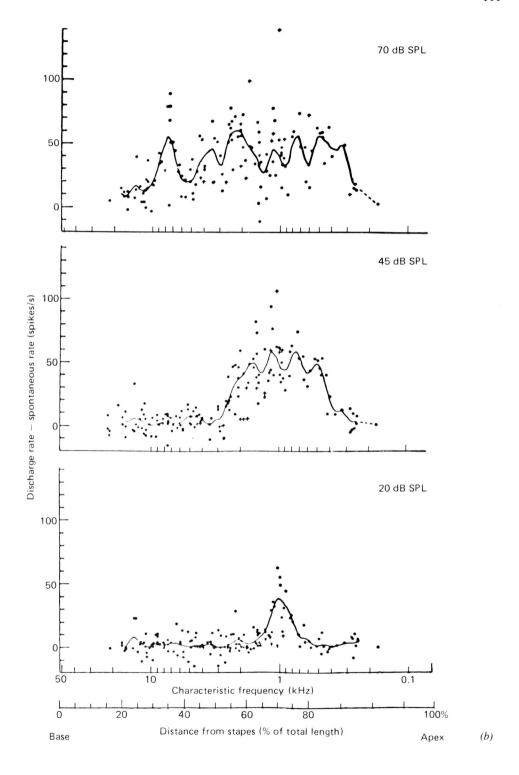

(b)

large, open circles. Thus, taking these results at face value, the neural filter bandwidths are more than adequate to account for the psychoacoustic frequency selectivity of the ear. (There are a number of difficulties in attempting to reconcile filter bandwidths derived from all the different psychoacoustic, animal behavioural and physiological techniques of measurement, but taken together they suggest that a value of about 10% for bandwidth – about one sixth of an octave – affords a reasonable description of the filtering ability of the cochlea.)

To a first approximation, therefore, the ear's psychoacoustic frequency selectivity is already determined at the level of the cochlea. The cochlea, therefore, is no mere microphone, but is instrumental in carrying out much of the most important function of frequency analysis. Without this we would not be able to hear speech clearly, or distinguish the individual instruments of an orchestra. In principle, the filtering ability of the cochlea produces a map of the distribution of energy at different frequencies in a complex sound into the degree of activity along the cochlear nerve fibre array. At low stimulus levels, therefore, the pattern of activity along the cochlear nerve fibre array will reflect the distribution of sound energy across the frequency spectrum. In *Figure 8.3* this is shown for single tones, but recently it has been beautifully demonstrated for speech sounds (Sachs and Kiang, 1968). *Figure 8.3* shows the distribution of activity in the cochlear nerve fibre array for 2 frequencies (8 kHz and 1 kHz). At low sound levels (20 dB SPL) the activity is restricted to a small number of fibres whose CFs coincide with the stimulus frequency. As the level of the stimulus is progressively increased, because of the overlap of the cochlear fibre FTCs, the activity spreads into more and more cochlear fibres of adjacent CFs, and so the active array expands. For low frequencies, e.g. 1 kHz, this presents a formidable problem, and the question arises as to how the upper levels of the auditory system are to determine that this activity represents that of a single tone. At higher frequencies, e.g. 8 kHz, the situation is better because of the extremely steep high-frequency cut-off of the FTCs (*Figure 8.1b*). Therefore an extremely sharp border between activity and inactivity is maintained, corresponding to the tone frequency. But again, it is not obvious how the higher levels of the auditory nervous system can use this information to distinguish whether there is more than one component in the acoustic signal. This is the so-called 'dynamic range problem' (Evans, 1978a, 1981), which is beyond the scope of this discussion, but which is receiving a great deal of attention from physiologists at the moment. It is possible that the frequencies in a complex sound at high stimulus levels may be conveyed either by a very small number of nerve fibres able to respond over a much wider dynamic range than the majority, or by the higher levels of the auditory nervous system being able to analyse in some way the fine time structure of the temporal patterning of the cochlear fibre discharges, or possibly both.

One question which has dominated a great deal of cochlear physiology in the last 20 years is how this extremely sharp tuning is achieved by the cochlea. Until very recently, measurements of the tuning of the basilar membrane had shown it to be much too broadly tuned to account for the sharp cochlear fibre tuning properties (Békésy, 1944; Johnstone, Taylor and Boyle, 1970; Rhode, 1971; Wilson and Johnstone, 1975). Thus, in *Figure 8.1b*, the curves representing measurements of basilar membrane vibration in the guinea-pig are plotted so as to be analogous with the cochlear fibre FTCs. The basilar membrane curves appear to be those of low pass filters. These, and other findings, suggested that in the cochlea we might have a two-stage filtering process: a first filter, that of the basilar membrane, followed by a hypothetical 'second filter' responsible for the sharp band-pass tuning properties of the cochlear fibres (Evans, 1972; Evans and Wilson, 1973). Some very recent (and unpublished) measurements of basilar membrane motion, however, suggest that the previous results may well describe what might be called the passive vibration characteristics of the basilar membrane. Under conditions where the measurement technique does not disturb the very delicate organ of Corti, much more sharply tuned responses have been obtained. These, and other results to be referred to later, suggest that the basilar membrane and organ of Corti may work together to form an active filter complex.

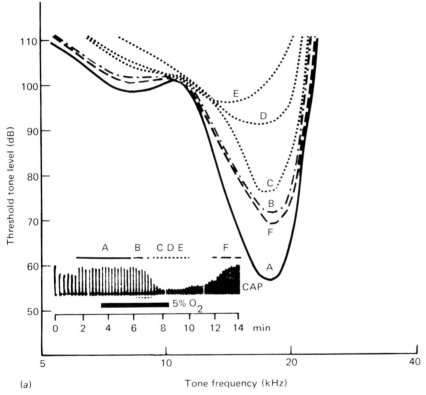

(a)

Figure 8.4a Reversible effects of hypoxia on the tuning of a single cochlear fibre in the cat. Inset shows time course of gross cochlear action potential (CAP) amplitude in response to click stimuli of constant amplitude (approximately 40 dB above threshold) presented every 10 s. The thick bar indicates the duration of reduction of inspired oxygen to 5%. The bars over the CAP record indicate the times during which the FTCs illustrated in the main figure were determined. (A) Control obtained before cochlear hypoxia developed (*see text*). (B to E) FTCs during development of cochlear hypoxia. (F) During recovery from hypoxia. Note loss and partial recovery of low-threshold, sharply tuned segment of FTC. (Modified from Evans, 1974b)

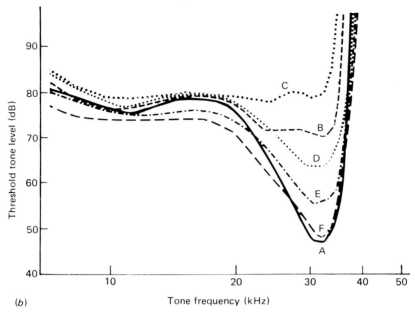

(b)

Tone frequency (kHz)

Figure 8.4b Reversible effects of frusemide (furosemide), a potent ototoxic diuretic, on FTC of cat cochlear fibre. Frusemide 20 mg was injected into the subclavian artery of the same side as the cochlea. (A) Control. (B, C) FTCs during action of frusemide on cochlea. Note loss of low-threshold segment of FTC. (D, E, F) Recovery. (Modified from Evans and Klinke, 1974).

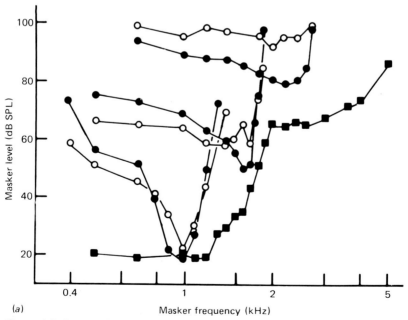

(a)

Masker frequency (kHz)

Figure 8.5 See caption on facing page

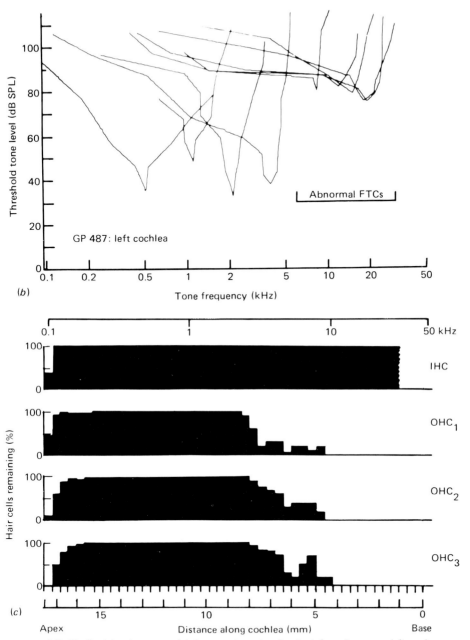

Figure 8.5 Similarities between (*a*) human 'psychophysical (psychoacoustic) tuning curves' in a patient with high frequency hearing loss and (*b*) physiological 'tuning curves' in a guinea-pig ear damaged by kanamycin. (*c*) Proportion of inner and outer hair cells remaining in the cochlea of the guinea-pig at the time of the physiological recording. All of the outer hair cells (OHC) are missing from the first 4–5 mm of the cochlea, the high-frequency end. The cochlear nerve tuning curves (*b*) have lost their sharp tuning in the region corresponding to the loss of outer hair cells. The 'psychoacoustic tuning curves' (*a*) are obtained by a tone-on-tone masking technique (*see text*). (Modified from Evans and Harrison, 1976; Wightman, McGee and Kramer, 1977)

An important discovery of the last 15 years relevant to this question is that the cochlear filtering mechanism is physiologically vulnerable. This means that alterations in the physiological condition of the cochlea can cause the normally sharp filtering properties to deteriorate. A variety of effects can cause reversible alteration in the cochlea's filtering. Thus, a short period of hypoxia (Evans, 1974a, 1974b; Robertson and Manley, 1974) or an intra-arterial injection of frusemide (furosemide) (Evans and Klinke, 1974) will cause, within the space of a few minutes, the cochlear fibre FTC to lose its low-threshold, sharply tuned tip and become high-threshold and broadly tuned (*Figures 8.4a and b*). If the physiological insult is short-lived, virtually complete recovery of the tuning can occur. Similar, but irreversible, effects have been shown to occur as a result of overexposure of the ear to sounds (Liberman and Kiang, 1978), and to the aminoglycoside antibiotics such as kanamycin (Kiang, Moxon and Levine, 1970; *Figure 8.5*). In these cases it is often the outer hair cells which are preferentially destroyed, and the changes in the FTCs noted in *Figure 8.4* occur for those fibres originating in the cochlear regions where the outer hair cells are missing. This is mapped out in *Figure 8.5* for the same guinea-pig cochlea from which the cochlear nerve FTCs were measured. While the inner hair cells appear to be intact (by light microscopical examination at least), the outer hair cells are missing from the basal half-turn (0–5 mm). The corresponding frequencies are about 10 to 15 kHz, and here the FTCs are high-threshold and blunt. (The significance of *Figure 8.5a* will be discussed later.) Findings such as these suggest that the normal sharp tuning of cochlear nerve fibres, most of which originate in the inner hair cells (Spoendlin, 1972), might be dependent upon the integrity of the outer hair cells. This apparently paradoxical situation has led to the suggestion that some form of interaction occurs between the inner and outer hair cells either at the mechanical, cellular, electrical or even neural level (Zwislocki and Sokolich, 1974; Evans, 1976). The latter possibility has been unequivocally excluded by the very recent microelectrode recordings from individual inner hair cells in the guinea-pig cochlea by Russell and Sellick (1978) (*Figure 8.6b*). Recording from the basal turn of the guinea-pig cochlea, these workers showed that inner hair cells produce an asymmetrical receptor potential reflecting the stimulus waveform (*Figure 8.6a*). At high frequencies the receptor potential is not able to 'follow' the stimulus waveform, and a d.c. potential remains. This receptor potential is as sharply tuned (*Figure 8.6b*) as the cochlear nerve fibre FTCs. Whatever the cochlear filtering mechanisms are, they must precede the generation of receptor potentials in the inner hair cells.

Another very recent and exciting finding relevant to this question of cochlear filtering is the demonstration that ears not only receive sounds, but under certain conditions can emit sounds (Kemp, 1978; Wilson, 1980). This acoustic emission can take two forms: an evoked emission, where a brief click or tone burst can evoke a brief emission, the so-called cochlear 'echo' (*Figure 8.7*), and a continuous spontaneous emission untriggered by an external stimulus. Much recent work suggests that this strange phenomenon may originate within the organ of Corti by mechanisms not understood. Very recently, the organ of Corti has been shown to contain contractile proteins, particularly actin (Flock, 1980). This leads to the highly speculative suggestion that the organ of Corti may be able to respond

117

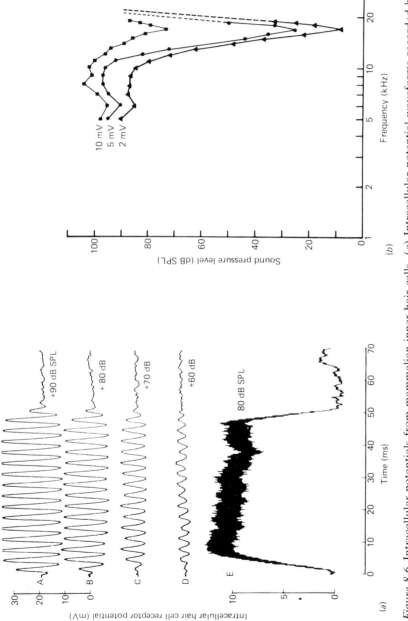

Figure 8.6 Intracellular potentials from mammalian inner hair cells. (*a*) Intracellular potential waveforms recorded by a microelectrode in an inner hair cell in the basal (high-frequency) turn of a guinea-pig. (A–D) Response to a tone burst of low frequency (300 Hz) and at different sound pressure levels. The waveform of the stimulus can be seen in the response (with distortion at high levels). (E) Response to a 3 kHz tone. Note small a.c. response superimposed upon a substantial (c. 12 mV) depolarizing potential (By courtesy of I. Russell and P. Sellick). (*b*) Variation in stimulus level required to keep d.c. receptor potential constant across frequency for three voltages (isovoltage frequency tuning curves). (Modified from Russell and Sellick, 1978)

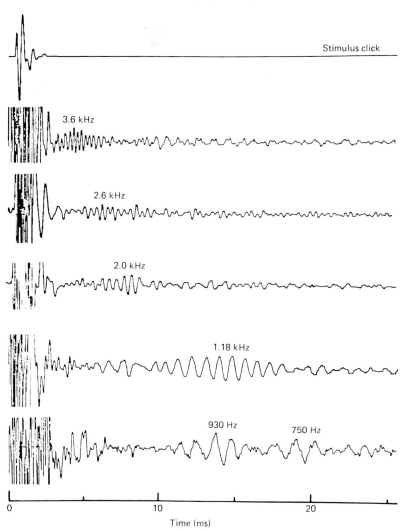

Figure 8.7 Evoked 'cochlear emissions'. Averaged responses to clicks recorded by a sensitive microphone in the ear canal of five human subjects. The first 3 ms shows averager overloaded by stimulus (top curve). Subjects were chosen to show a wide range of response frequencies and the corresponding change of latency. (From Wilson, 1980, courtesy of the Editor and Publishers, *Hearing Research*)

mechanically to incoming sounds. Since the cochlear emission phenomenon is physiologically vulnerable and has a number of other features related to the sharp tuning of cochlear nerve fibres, it has been suggested that the phenomenon may be bound up with the cochlear frequency selective mechanism (Kemp and Chum, 1980). This would mean that the cochlear 'micromechanics', i.e. the mechanical properties of the basilar membrane–organ of Corti complex, are not passive, but active in the sense of requiring energy for normal sharp tuning function, and possibly involving the active generation of vibration. It is conceivable that such a mechanism could achieve a high degree of sensitivity and tuning by means of 'positive feedback' whereby a mechanical response is generated by the organ of Corti in phase with the incoming signal. This must remain in the realms of speculation, however, until further information on these phenomena becomes available. Yet, taken together, all the recent data do suggest that the cochlea can no longer be considered to have passive mechanics, but that the activity of the hair cells (the hypothetical 'second filter') must be an integral part of the cochlear 'micromechanics' and be the source of energy input to the filtering process. There is even accumulating evidence that the active mechanical properties of the cochlea can be controlled by stimulation of the efferent nerve supply to the cochlea (Mountain, 1980). Thus it is possible that the mechanical stiffness properties of the hairs or hair cells could be controlled by efferent 'tone'. Again, the situation here is paradoxical: the great majority of cochlear efferents in mammals end upon the outer hair cells, whereas the majority of afferent nerve fibres originate from the inner hair cells (Spoendlin, 1972). Presumably the micromechanics of the cochlea must depend on the physical integrity and mechanical properties of the cellular elements within the organ of Corti, particularly the outer hair cells.

ANIMAL MODELS OF COCHLEAR HEARING LOSS AND TINNITUS

Cochlear hearing loss

It will be clear from the above that the cochlear filtering mechanisms are extremely vulnerable to physiological insult. Overexposure to noise, reduction in the oxygen supply to the cochlea, and exposure to loop diuretics (e.g. frusemide) and aminoglycosides (e.g. kanamycin) all produce a deterioration in the filtering characteristics which, if prolonged, becomes permanent (*see Figure 8.5*). Similar effects are obtained as a result of surgical interference with the cochlea (*see Figure 8.1b*; curves A–D), haemorrhage, etc. In other words, all modifications in cochlear function so far studied have one common end result: deterioration in the tuning properties of the cochlear nerve fibres.

This means that in human cochlear pathology we should expect an identical deterioration in the frequency selectivity of the cochlea. Obviously we cannot study this directly; hence there has been considerable interest in the last 10 years in the study of 'animal models' of hearing loss, and in extrapolations from these animal models to clinical findings. The animal models suggest that for the types of cochlear pathology mentioned above the chief physiological change is a deterioration in frequency selectivity. Interestingly, virtually no changes in the temporal discharge patterns of cochlear nerve fibres have been observed (Harrison and Evans, 1978). It should be mentioned that no animal model of cochlear hydrops, in which it is likely that changes in the temporal discharge patterns may be found, has yet been studied.

If the frequency selectivity function of the auditory system is already largely determined at the cochlear nerve level, then we should expect, under conditions of cochlear pathology, deterioration in this ability. This has been recently demonstrated to occur by a variety of techniques. Of the psychoacoustic techniques, the most readily understood (although possibly the most difficult to apply) is that of the 'psychoacoustic tuning curve' (*see Figure 8.5a*). These psychoacoustic tuning curves are obtained by plotting the frequencies and intensities at which a second tone will mask a tone of constant frequency and intensity. The shape of the psychoacoustic tuning curves resembles that of cochlear fibre FTCs in normal ears, supporting the statement that the ear's psychoacoustic frequency selectivity is already largely determined at the cochlear nerve level. Under conditions of cochlear pathology, however, the psychoacoustic tuning curves lose their sharply tuned low-threshold tip and become as blunt as the physiological tuning curves obtained in animal models of cochlear hearing loss (*see Figure 8.5*). Other psychoacoustic methods are more easily applied in the clinic and involve, for example, the masking of a test tone by comb-filtered noise, i.e. noise stimuli having alternating peaks and valleys in the spectrum (Pick, Evans and Wilson, 1977). These measurements allow determination of the filtering bandwidths of the ear at different frequencies. *Figure 8.8* shows the results of such measurements at four frequencies for a number of patients with unilateral cochlear hearing loss, mainly Ménière's disease. Generally speaking, the greater the hearing loss, the greater the deterioration in frequency selectivity, in other words, the wider the tuning bandwidth. This is in agreement with the findings in animal models of cochlear pathology. It is clear, however, that there is a large variation from point to point, representing individual ear differences. *Figure 8.8*, for example, shows one patient measured at 2 kHz with a modest hearing loss of about 30 dB, yet with one of the largest filter bandwidths (1.5 kHz). This means that there is not necessarily a direct relationship between loss of sensitivity (threshold elevation) and deterioration in frequency selectivity, although on average this is the case. Deterioration in frequency selectivity can therefore be used as a sensitive test of damage to the cochlear function, at least in certain individuals (Pick and Evans, 1980), and is a direct measure of the expected loss in auditory function. A number of laboratories are therefore investigating the value of more selective and specialized tests such as these for the diagnosis and assessment of patients with cochlear hearing loss.

Another approach is to use the auditory evoked potentials. Using electrocochleography and simple masking techniques (Harrison, Aran and Erre, 1981), it is possible to obtain so-called 'gross cochlear action potential tuning curves', which resemble approximately the tuning curves of individual cochlear nerve fibres. Under conditions of cochlear pathology in both animals and man, these gross cochlear action potential tuning curves show a similar deterioration in shape to that shown in *Figure 8.5*.

These findings from animal models of cochlear pathology are relevant to our understanding of the changes in auditory processing of diagnostic importance, namely the recruitment of loudness and the intelligibility of speech.

Recruitment of loudness can be simply accounted for by the changes observed in animal models in the properties of cochlear fibres. Two possible factors can be identified from these. The first is the change in frequency selectivity of the cochlear

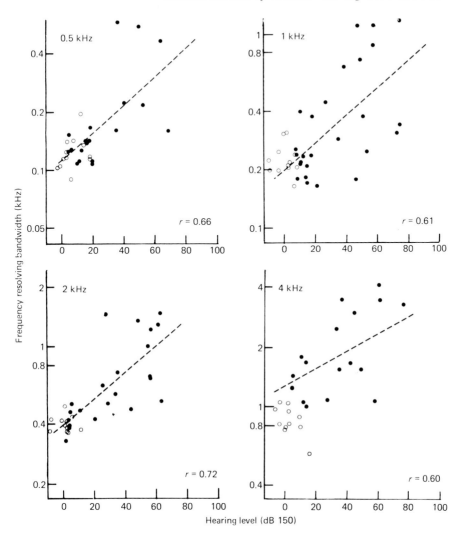

Figure 8.8 Relationship between level of hearing loss and filter bandwidths calculated from comb-filtered noise measurements for normal subjects and patients with cochlear hearing loss. Each plot displays the bandwidths computed from determinations of frequency resolving power at the frequency indicated. (○) Normal ears (including normal ears of patients); (●) affected ears; (–––) regression line from patient data. (From Pick, Evans and Wilson, 1977, courtesy of the Publishers, *Psychophysics and Physiology of Hearing*)

fibres (*Figure 8.9a*). If loudness is related to the number of cochlear nerve fibres that are active, then, in the normal cochlea, it will grow slowly at first, corresponding to the slow recruitment of cochlear nerve fibres of adjacent CFs having sharply tuned tips. At higher sound levels, growth will be more rapid because the signal will cross into a larger number of FTCs by virtue of their low frequency 'tails'. In contrast, in pathological fibres, where the low-threshold sharply tuned tips are missing, once the signal reaches the threshold of the FTCs it will recruit adjacent fibres at a very rapid rate (Evans, 1975b, 1975c).

The second factor may be the rate of increase in discharge rate with stimulus level. In both acute (Evans, 1975b; Evans and Borerwe, 1982) and chronic (Harrison and Evans, 1979) pathological conditions of the cochlea, the rate at which the cochlear fibre's discharge rate increases with stimulus level is substantially steeper than in normal fibres (*Figure 8.9b*). In other words, the dynamic range of pathological cochlear fibres is less, on average, than that of normal cochlear fibres. If the loudness of a sound depends on the rate of cochlear fibre discharges as well as on the number of fibres active, these two factors will combine to produce an

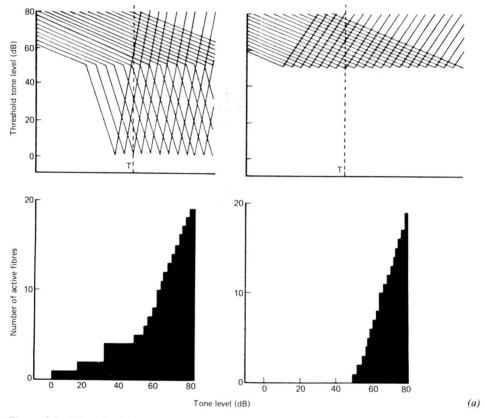

Figure 8.9a Hypothetical processes underlying recruitment. Schematic diagrams illustrating rate of growth in number of active cochlear fibres with tone stimulus level in normal (*left*) and abnormal (*right*) cochleas. (– – –) Tone frequency indicated at T. (*Top*) Sharply tuned FTCs of single cochlear fibres in normal cochlea; high-threshold, broadly tuned FTCs of abnormal cochlea (as in *Figures 8.4 and 8.5*). (*Bottom*) Growth in number of active fibres with increasing tone level, as a result of the difference in sharpness and threshold of the cochlear fibre FTCs in normal (*left*) and abnormal (*right*) cochleas. Each new fibre is added to the active group as the tone level crosses its FTC. The scales in each plot are arbitrary. In the case of the tone intensity scales in particular, the dB values are given purely for convenience in relating the upper and lower plots, and are not intended to represent absolute threshold values. (Modified from Evans, 1975b)

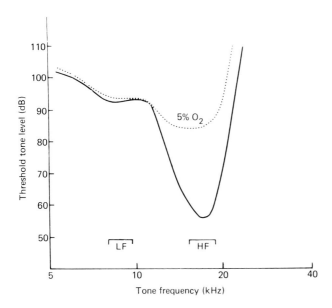

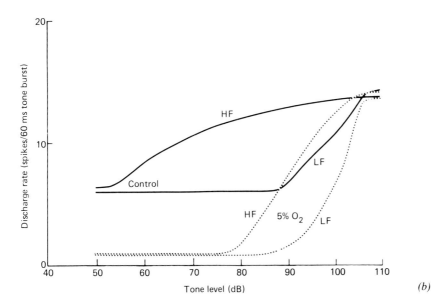

Figure 8.9b Effect of hypoxia on cochlear nerve discharge rate versus tone in relation to changes in the FTC. (*Top*) FTCs of single cochlear fibre in cat before (———) and during (.....) hypoxia. Conditions similar to those in *Figure 8.4a*. (*Bottom*) Discharge rates of the cochlear fibre as a function of the relative tone level, averaged over a band of low frequencies (LF), and a band of frequencies about the CF (HF) before (———) and during (.....) hypoxia, i.e. corresponding to the FTCs shown above. Note, in the control case, the greater steepness of the low frequency (LF) function in comparison with that at the CF (HF) and the steepening of the latter under hypoxia (*see text*). (Modified from Evans, 1975b)

abnormally rapid rise in loudness with stimulus level, pathognomonic of cochlear hearing loss. The same arguments apply to the growth of the amplitude of the gross cochlear action potential measured by electrocochleography, which is found to be steeper (termed 'recruiting') in cases of cochlear pathology (Aran, 1971).

The second aspect of auditory processing predicted to be affected by cochlear pathology on the basis of these animal studies is the processing of speech. Deterioration in speech intelligibility would be expected to result from several aspects of the deterioration in physiological frequency selectivity. Moreover, because the deterioration occurs at the level of the cochlea, which is responsible for the ear's frequency selectivity, it is unlikely that the higher levels of the auditory system will be capable of overcoming these deficiencies in peripheral processing. Hence linear amplification of sounds by the current generation of hearing aids could not be expected to compensate for these changes. This goes some way towards explaining why linear amplification *per se* is of little value to patients with moderate to severe cochlear hearing losses. It should be emphasized, however, that deterioration in frequency selectivity is not likely to be the only factor involved: the temporal coding of speech is also affected in a way not at all understood in physiological terms (Evans, 1982). One consequence of deterioration in physiological frequency selectivity would be a 'blurring' of the neural representation of the frequencies in speech sound (*Figure 8.10*). Speech sounds contain a number of concentrations of energy at certain frequencies, called formant frequencies (*Figure 8.10a*). In the normal cochlea (at least at low to moderate sound levels) these concentrations of sound energy could be expected to be represented in peaks of activity along the cochlear nerve fibre array from the apex to the base of the cochlea (*Figure 8.10b*). Under pathological conditions of the cochlea, however, where the tuning of the individual cochlear nerve fibres has become blunt, this would be expected to 'smear out' the peaks of activity (*Figure 8.10c*). Under these conditions, no further processing by the upper levels of the auditory system can easily compensate for the lost information.

In addition, other factors arising from the deterioration of the cochlea's frequency selectivity contribute to a deterioration in speech intelligibility. Because of the loss of the sharply tuned low-threshold tip of the tuning curves, one would expect a pathologically increased upward spread of masking, leading to increased masking of the less intense higher frequency formants by the more intense lower frequency formants. This has been demonstrated in patients with cochlear hearing loss (Danaher and Pickett, 1975). In addition, sharp filtering normally favours the ability of the auditory system to extract signals in the presence of background noise. Deterioration in filtering will reduce this ability and could account for the increased susceptibility of the cochlear-impaired ear to masking of signals by background noise. Finally, the fact that interaural processing mechanisms responsible for accurate location of sound sources in space may depend on normal frequency selective mechanisms (Scharf, 1978) may explain why patients with cochlear hearing loss experience difficulties in understanding speech in a 'cocktail party' environment. Under these conditions the peripheral auditory mechanism appears unable to avoid the masking of one voice by another, which the normal ear can do if the two sound sources are separated in space. With the possible exception of the

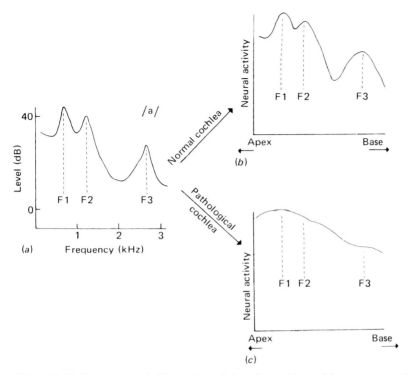

Figure 8.10 Diagrammatic illustration of the effect of loss of frequency resolution on speech perception. (*a*) Energy spectrum of a whispered vowel (/a/). (*b*) Diagram showing how this vowel might be encoded by the normal cochlea. (*c*) Hypothetical neural mapping of the expected representation in the pathological cochlea. F1, F2, F3 = Formant frequencies (*see text*). (From Pick and Evans, 1982, courtesy of the Publishers, *High Technology Aids for Disabled People*)

last effect, which appears to be relatively independent of threshold elevation (Pick and Evans, 1980), the changes in frequency selectivity observed in animal models of cochlear pathology are most obvious with threshold elevations above about 40 dB (Evans, 1978b). This would appear to correlate with the observation that no substantial loss of speech discrimination ability occurs until the hearing threshold is elevated to some 30 to 40 dB above normal (Hood and Poole, 1971). Changes in the cut-off slopes of the cochlear fibre tuning curves, however, follow elevations in threshold more closely, particularly for the low-frequency cut-off. This would therefore be likely to be manifest in early signs of recruitment.

Animal models of tinnitus

In the last 2 or 3 years, efforts have been directed at setting up valid animal models of human tinnitus. A major problem has been to devise a behavioural index which would show that an animal is experiencing tinnitus. Two ways round this problem have been explored (Evans, Wilson and Borerwe, 1981).

The first is to use salicylate in doses which are sufficient to raise blood levels to those associated with tinnitus in man (Mongan *et al.*, 1973). This has been done in a number of anaesthetized cats (Evans and Borerwe, 1982; Evans, Wilson and Borerwe, 1981). Salicylates, like the other ototoxic agents, produce elevation in threshold and reduction in the tuning of cochlear fibres (Evans and Borerwe, 1982). The question was: would salicylates produce the reduction in spontaneous discharge activity observed, as a rule, in the case of the other ototoxic agents?

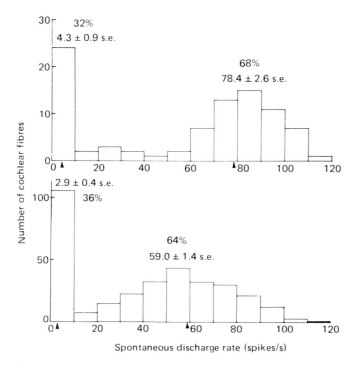

Figure 8.11 Distribution of spontaneous activity of cochlear nerve fibres following administration of salicylate compared with that from normal cat cochleas. Data were obtained from 88 fibres in a single cat after salicylate (*top*), and 333 fibres in six cats with normal cochleas (*bottom*). Note bimodal distribution of spontaneous activity in both cases, the means of each subpopulation being indicated by the values above, and the arrows below, each histogram. Note the shift in distribution of spontaneous activity of the high-spontaneous-rate sub-population following salicylate. (From Evans, Wilson and Borerwe, 1981, courtesy of the publishers, *Tinnitus*)

Figure 8.11 shows the distribution of spontaneous discharge rates of a large number of cochlear fibres in an animal with high blood levels of salicylate, compared with the distribution of spontaneous discharge rates of fibres in normal ears. In both situations the distribution of spontaneous discharge rates is bimodal: about one-third of fibres have spontaneous discharge rates below about 20 spikes/s, the majority being virtually silent, whereas about two-thirds have a wide range of discharge rates, extending up to about 120 spikes/s. The normal mean of the higher spontaneous discharge rate population is about 60 spikes/s. Under salicylates, however, the mean of the high spontaneous rate population shifts upwards, i.e. in the opposite direction to that normally encountered in animal studies of the effects of ototoxic agents. This may well be a physiological correlate of salicylate-induced tinnitus. The only other report in the literature of an increase in spontaneous discharge rate following cochlear pathology is that by Liberman and Kiang (1978), who observed this phenomenon in a minority of cats examined about one month following noise overstimulation. This, again, may be the correlate of tinnitus in cases of noise overstimulation.

Accompanying the increases in spontaneous discharge rate in salicylate poisoning are alterations in the temporal discharge patterns of cochlear fibres (Evans and Borerwe, 1982; Evans, Wilson and Borerwe, 1981). Whether these are relevant to the perception of tinnitus is unknown.

Following clinical reports of suppression of tinnitus by means of electrical stimulation of the cochlea, analogous experiments have recently been carried out in animal models (Evans and Borerwe (1982). A consistent finding is that positive currents directed into the round window can reduce the spontaneous discharge activity of all cochlear fibres so far examined (*Figure 8.12*). This again lends support to the hypothesis that tinnitus of cochlear origin is normally associated with an increase in the spontaneous discharge rate of the cochlear nerve fibres.

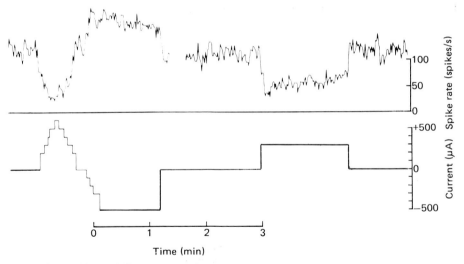

Figure 8.12 Effect of direct current into round window on mean spontaneous activity oi a normal cochlear fibre (characteristic frequency 23 kHz). Current strength is indicated in µA, positive to round window (+); negative (−). (From Evans and Borerwe, 1982, courtesy of the Editor and Publishers, *British Journal of Audiology*)

A second animal model of tinnitus that has recently been studied is that of a continuous, tonal emission in a guinea-pig (Evans, Wilson and Borerwe, 1981). This emission had a number of characteristics in common with that recorded in human subjects (Wilson, 1980): it could be recorded as an acoustic signal in the ear canal; its amplitude and frequency were affected by changes in the stiffness of the middle ear system; and it could be synchronized by tones of neighbouring frequency and suppressed by tones of higher frequency. The levels of the continuous emission and the synchronizing and suppressing tones were analogous to those recorded in man. In the animal model, however, it was possible to demonstrate that the emission could be recorded as an electrical signal from the round window (Evans, Wilson and Borerwe, 1981). It was also possible to demonstrate that the tonal emission was not likely to be generated by the middle ear: it was unaffected by muscle-paralyzing agents and by section of the tendon of the stapedius muscle. Furthermore, it could be substantially attenuated in the ear canal by changes in the stiffness of the middle ear system, without significant change in the amplitude of the round window recorded signal. Its latency (4 ms) was also too short for the middle ear muscles to be involved. The sensitivity of the emission both to acoustic trauma and to hypoxia indicated that it was as physiologically vulnerable as the tuning of cochlear nerve fibres. All the evidence therefore suggests that the origin of this spontaneous emission is some form of metabolically labile mechanical disturbance within the cochlea itself, of the kind discussed above in connection with the 'cochlear echo' phenomenon. Measurements on human subjects suggest that this form of tinnitus, associated with a recordable signal in the ear canal, is likely to be restricted to the category of so-called 'physiological tinnitus' (Wilson and Sutton, 1981). How far it is representative of the types of tinnitus encountered clinically is currently under study.

Acknowledgements

I am grateful to Dr D. J. Parker for making helpful comments on the manuscript, and to Mr R. Brunt for technical assistance.

References

Aran, J. M. (1971) The electrocochleogram: recent results in children and in some pathological cases. *Archiv für Klinische und Experimentelle Ohren-, Nasen und Kehlkopfeilkunde*, **198**, 128–141

Békésy, G. von (1944) Über die mechanische Frequenzanalyse in der Schnecke verschiedener Tiere. *Akustika Zeitschrift*, **9**, 3–11

Danaher, E. M. and Pickett, J. M. (1975) Some masking effects produced by low-frequency vowel formants in persons with sensorineural hearing loss. *Journal of Speech and Hearing Research*, **18**, 261–271

Evans, E. F. (1972) The frequency response and other properties of single fibres in the guinea pig cochlear nerve. *Journal of Physiology*, **226**, 263–287

Evans, E. F. (1974a) The effects of hypoxia on the tuning of single cochlear nerve fibres. *Journal of Physiology*, **238**, 65–67P

Evans, E. F. (1974b) Auditory frequency selectivity and the cochlear nerve. In *Facts and Models in Hearing*, edited by E. Zwicker and E. Terhardt, pp. 118–129. Heidelberg: Springer-Verlag

Evans, E. F. (1975a) The cochlear nerve and cochlear nucleus. In *Handbook of Sensory Physiology*, **5,** Part 2, edited by W. D. Keidel and W. D. Neff. pp. 1–108. Heidelberg: Springer-Verlag

Evans, E. F. (1975b) Normal and abnormal functioning of the cochlear nerve. In *Sound Reception in Mammals* (Symposium of the Zoological Society of London, No. 37), edited by R. J. Bench, A. Pye and J. D. Pye, pp. 133–165. London: Academic Press

Evans, E. F. (1975c) The sharpening of cochlear frequency selectivity in the normal and abnormal cochlea. *Audiology*, **14,** 419–442

Evans, E. F. (1976) Temporal sensorineural hearing losses and 8th nerve changes. In *Effects of Noise on Hearing: Critical Issues*, edited by D. Henderson, R. P. Hamernik, D. S. Dosanjh and J. H. Mills, pp. 199–221. New York: Raven Press

Evans, E. F. (1978a) Place and time coding of frequency in the peripheral auditory system: some physiological pros and cons. *Audiology*, **17,** 369–420

Evans, E. F. (1978b) Peripheral auditory processing in normal and abnormal ears: physiological considerations for attempts to compensate for auditory deficits by acoustic and electrical prostheses. In *Sensorineural Hearing Impairment and Hearing Aids*, edited by C. Ludvigsen and J. Barfod, pp. 9–44. *Scandinavian Audiology*, Suppl. **6**

Evans, E. F. (1981) The dynamic range problem: place and time coding at the level of cochlear nerve and nucleus. In *Neuronal Mechanisms of Hearing*, edited by J. Syka and L. Aitken, pp. 69–85. New York: Plenum Press

Evans, E. F. (1982) Breakdown of hearing mechanisms in hearing disorders. In *Hearing Science and Hearing Disorders*, edited by M. Lutman and M. P. Haggard. London: Academic Press

Evans, E. F. and Borerwe, T. A. (1982) Ototoxic effects of salicylates on the responses of single cochlear nerve fibres and on cochlear potentials. *British Journal of Audiology*, **16,** 101–108

Evans, E. F. and Harrison, R. V. (1976) Correlation between outer hair cell damage and deterioration of cochlear nerve tuning properties in the guinea pig. *Journal of Physiology*, **256,** 43–44P

Evans, E. F. and Klinke, R. (1974) Reversible effects of cyanide and furosemide on the tuning of single cochlear fibres. *Journal of Physiology*, **242,** 129–131P

Evans, E. F. and Wilson, J. P. (1973) Frequency selectivity of the cochlea. In *Basic Mechanisms in Hearing*, edited by A. R. Moller, pp. 519–551. New York: Academic Press

Evans, E. F., Wilson, J. P. and Borerwe, T. A. (1981) Animal models of tinnitus. In *Tinnitus* (CIBA Foundation Symposium 85), edited by D. Evered and G. Lawrenson, pp. 108–129. London: Pitman Medical

Flock, A. (1980) Contractile proteins in hair cells. *Hearing Research*, **2,** 411–412

Harrison, R. V., Aran, J. M. and Erre, J.-P. (1981) AP tuning curves from normal and pathological human and guinea pig cochleas. *Journal of the Acoustical Society of America*, **69,** 1374–1385

Harrison, R. V. and Evans, E. F. (1978) Some aspects of temporal coding by single cochlear fibres from regions of cochlear hair cell degeneration in the guinea pig. *Archives of Otorhinolaryngology*, **224,** 71–78

Harrison, R. V. and Evans, E. F. (1979) Cochlear fibre responses in guinea pigs with well-defined cochlear lesions. In *Models of the Auditory System and Related Signal Processing Techniques*, edited by M. Hoke and E. de Boer, pp. 83–92. *Scandinavian Audiology*, Suppl. **9**

Hood, J. D. and Poole, J. P. (1971) Speech audiometry in conductive and sensorineural hearing loss. *Sound*, **5**, 30–38

Johnstone, B. M., Taylor, K. J. and Boyle, A. J. (1970) Mechanics of the guinea pig cochlea. *Journal of the Acoustical Society of America*, **47**, 504–509

Kemp, D. T. (1978) Stimulated acoustic emissions from the human auditory system. *Journal of the Acoustical Society of America*, **64**, 1386–1391

Kemp, D. T. and Chum, R. (1980) Properties of the generator of stimulated acoustic emissions. *Hearing Research*, **2**, 213–232

Kiang, N. Y.-s., Moxon, E. C. and Levine, R. A. (1970) Auditory nerve activity in cats with normal and abnormal cochleas. In *Sensorineural Hearing Loss*, edited by G. E. W. Wolstenholme and J. Knight. London: Churchill

Kim, D. O. and Molnar, C. E. (1979) A population study of cochlear nerve fibres: comparison of spatial distributions of average rate and phase-locking measures of responses to single tones. *Journal of Neurophysiology*, **42**, 16–30

Liberman, M. C. L. and Kiang, N. Y.-s. (1978) Acoustic trauma in cats. *Acta Oto-Laryngologica* (Suppl.), **358**

Mongan, E., Kelly, P., Nies, K., Porter, W. W. and Paulus, H. F. (1973) Tinnitus as an indication of therapeutic serum salicylate levels. *Journal of the American Medical Association*, **226**, 142–145

Mountain, D. C. (1980) Changes in endolymphatic potential and crossed olivo-cochlear bundle stimulation alter basilar membrane mechanics. *Science*, **210**, 71–72

Pick, G. F. and Evans, E. F. (1980) Frequency resolution in patients with difficulty in speech perception but with normal audiograms. Paper presented at Meeting of British Society of Audiology, Nottingham, July 7th

Pick, G. F. and Evans, E. F. (1982) Strategies for high-technology hearing aids to compensate for hearing impairment of cochlear origin. In *High Technology Aids for Disabled People*, edited by W. J. Perkins. London: Butterworths (in press)

Pick, G. F., Evans, E. F. and Wilson, J. P. (1977) Frequency resolution of patients with hearing loss of cochlear origin. In *Psychophysics and Physiology of Hearing*, edited by E. F. Evans and J. P. Wilson, pp. 273–281. London: Academic Press

Pickles, J. O. (1975) Normal critical bands in the cat. *Acta Oto-Laryngologica*, **80**, 245–254

Rhode, W. S. (1971) Observations of the vibration of the basilar membrane in squirrel monkeys using the Mossbauer technique. *Journal of the Acoustical Society of America*, **49**, 1218–1231

Robertson, D. and Manley, G. A. (1974) Manipulation of frequency analysis in the cochlear ganglion of the guinea pig. *Journal of Comparative Physiology*, **91**, 363–375

Rose, J. E., Kitzes, L. M., Gibson, M. M. and Hind, J. E. (1974) Observations on phase-sensitive neurons of anteroventral cochlear nucleus of the cat: nonlinearity of cochlear output. *Journal of Neurophysiology*, **37**, 218–253

Russell, I. J. and Sellick, P. M. (1978) Intracellular studies of hair cells in the mammalian cochlea. *Journal of Physiology*, **284**, 261–290

Sachs, M. B. and Kiang, N. Y.-s. (1968) Two-tone inhibition in auditory nerve fibres. *Journal of the Acoustical Society of America*, **43**, 1120–1128

Sachs, M. B. and Young, E. D. (1979) Encoding of steady-state vowels in the auditory nerve: representation in terms of discharge rate. *Journal of the Acoustical Society of America*, **66**, 470–479

Scharf, B. (1978) Comparison of normal and impaired hearing. II. Frequency analysis, speech perception. In *Sensorineural Hearing Impairment and Hearing Aids*, edited by C. Ludvigsen and J. Barfod. *Scandinavian Audiology* Suppl. **6**, 81–103

Spoendlin, H. (1972) Innervation densities of the cochlea. *Acta Otolaryngologica (Stockholm)*, **73**, 235–248

Wightman, F., McGee, T. and Kramer, M. (1977) Factors influencing frequency selectivity in normal and hearing-impaired listeners. In *Psychophysics and Physiology of Hearing*, edited by E. F. Evans and J. P. Wilson, pp. 25–306. London: Academic Press

Wilson, J. P. (1980) Evidence for a cochlear origin for acoustic re-emissions, threshold fine-structure and tonal tinnitus. *Hearing Research*, **2**, 233–252

Wilson, J. P. and Sutton, G. J. (1981) Acoustic correlates of tonal tinnitus. In *Tinnitus* (CIBA Foundation Symposium 85), edited by D. Evered and G. Lawrenson, pp. 82–100. London: Pitman Medical

Wilson, J. P. and Johnstone, J. R. (1975) Basilar membrane and middle-ear vibration in guinea pig measured by capacitive probe. *Journal of the Acoustical Society of America*, **57**, 705–723

Young, E. D. and Sachs, M. B. (1979) Representation of steady-state vowels in the temporal aspects of the discharge patterns of populations of auditory nerve fibers. *Journal of the Acoustical Society of America*, **66**, 1381–1403

Zwislocki, J. J. and Sokolich, W. G. (1974) Neuro-mechanical frequency analysis in the cochlea. In *Facts and Models in Hearing*, edited by E. Zwicker and E. Terhardt, pp. 107–117. Berlin: Springer-Verlag

9
Auditory evoked responses
Derald E. Brackmann, Weldon A. Selters and
Manuel Don

During the past 10 years, electric response audiometry (ERA), particularly
brain-stem audiometry, has become an important clinical tool. In this course the
basic principles of electric response audiometry are reviewed. We then describe the
various techniques, emphasizing their clinical applications.

BASIC CONCEPTS OF ELECTRIC RESPONSE AUDIOMETRY

The aim of electric response audiometry is to record the potentials that arise in the
auditory system as a result of sound stimulation. The basic principles of recording
the electrical potentials from the auditory system are the same regardless of the
potential that is of particular interest. The recording is made difficult by the fact
that the potentials generated in the auditory system are minute in comparison with
the background of electrical impulses from other parts of the body (brain, heart and
muscles). The development of the average response computer has made it practical
to record these potentials in the clinical setting.

The apparatus for electric response audiometry is shown in simplified form as a
block diagram in *Figure 9.1* The stimulus is an acoustic impulse of very short
duration, termed a click, tone pip or tone burst. This brief stimulus produces a
synchronized discharge in the auditory system. The stimulus is attenuated and then
presented to the test ear through either a free-field loudspeaker or a headphone.
Depending on the technique employed, the active electrode is applied to the ear
lobe, mastoid prominence, ear canal, promontory or scalp vertex. An appropriate
reference electrode is also applied. The minute signal which these electrodes pick
up is first differentially amplified in a preamplifier and then further enlarged in an
amplifier before being delivered to the averaging computer.

The average response computer consists of a series of memory units, each
receiving information a fraction of a second later than the one just before it. We
like to think of each point as a small calculator capable of addition and subtraction.

The computer is triggered to begin its sequential process of analysis each time a

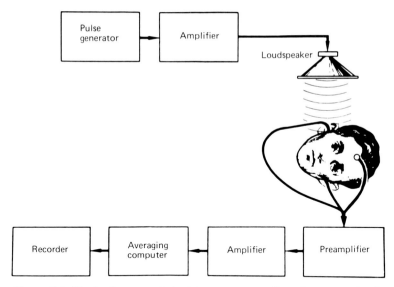

Figure 9.1 Block diagram of electric response audiometry apparatus (*see text for details*)

stimulus is delivered to the ear. The signal is said to be time-locked to the averager. In other words, the response repeatedly occurs in the same group of memory locations. In this way the potentials from the auditory system that singly would be impossible to identify are extracted from the background noise, which is reduced by the averaging. The averaged response is then transferred to permanent recording paper for analysis.

The basic principles for recording are the same in all electric response audiometry. The techniques vary depending on the response to be measured.

AUDITORY EVOKED POTENTIALS

The most important auditory evoked potentials, their probable sites of generation and typical latencies are outlined below.

(1) Cochlea (hair cells)
  Cochlear microphonic
  Summating potential

(2) Auditory nerve
  Eighth nerve action potential (wave I) 2.0 ms

(3) Brain stem
  Wave II – cochlear nucleus 3.0 ms
  Wave III – superior olive 4.1 ms
  Wave IV – lateral lemniscus 5.3 ms
  Wave V – inferior colliculus 5.9 ms
  Frequency following response – unknown
  Slow negative 10 (SN-10) – unknown 10.0 ms

(4) Middle responses (auditory cortex)
   N_o – 8 to 10 ms (variable)
   P_o – 13 ms
   N_a – 22 ms
   P_a – 34 ms
   N_b – 44 ms

(5) Vertex potential (auditory cortex)
   P_1 – 50 ms (variable)
   N_1 – 90 ms
   P_2 – 180 ms
   N_2 – 250 ms
   Sustained cortical potential
   Late positive component
   Contingent negative variation

In considering these responses it is important to point out that the measurements obtained from ERA methods are generally not measures of hearing *per se*. Hearing is a perceptual process that involves the entire auditory system and cannot be measured in terms of electric responses unless those responses can be shown to relate directly to perception. The clinical value of ERA lies in the correlation of electrical responses with auditory pathology and/or performance.

TYPES OF ELECTRIC RESPONSE AUDIOMETRY

Three techniques for recording the auditory evoked potentials have been described: electrocochleography (ECoG), auditory brain-stem response audiometry (ABR), and cortical electric response audiometry. A comparison of these techniques is presented in *Table 9.1*.

Table 9.1 Comparison of techniques of electric response audiometry

	Electrode	Effect of anesthesia	Portion of auditory system tested	Reliability
Electrocochleography	Promontory	None	Peripheral	Excellent
Auditory brain-stem response audiometry	Surface	None	Brain stem	Good
Cortical evoked response audiometry	Surface	Marked	Entire	Fair

Electrocochleography

Electrocochleography is the measurement of the potentials arising within the cochlea and the auditory nerve: cochlear microphonic, summating potential and eighth nerve action potential. In most cases a needle electrode is placed through the tympanic membrane on to the bone of the promontory to make these recordings.

Electrocochleography is the most accurate of the electric response audiometric techniques by virtue of the close proximity of the electrode to the generator sites. Accuracy is also enhanced because the peripheral auditory system is unaffected by sedation or even general anesthesia.

An obvious disadvantage of this technique is the requirement for tympanic membrane penetration. Another disadvantage is that it measures only the response of the most peripheral portion of the auditory system and therefore cannot be equated with hearing as such. Although relatively rare, there are cases in which the cochlea and auditory nerve function normally, but brain-stem or central defects produce hearing loss.

Auditory brain-stem response audiometry

Auditory brain-stem response audiometry uses surface electrodes to measure the potentials arising in the auditory nerve and brain-stem structures. The active electrode is placed on the scalp vertex, and the reference electrode is attached to the mastoid prominence of the test ear. The opposite mastoid is used as a ground. The events that occur during the first 10 ms following sound stimulation are recorded.

The advantage of auditory brain-stem response audiometry is that, because surface electrodes are used, anesthesia is not required. In practice, however, either basal narcosis or anesthesia is often required in children in order to prevent excessive movement which interferes with accurate recordings. Auditory brain-stem response audiometry, like electrocochleography, is not influenced by basal narcosis or general anesthesia.

Cortical electric response audiometry

Cortical electric response audiometry involves the measurement of the potentials that arise in the auditory system above the brain stem (the middle and slow potentials). The electrode configuration is the same as for auditory brain-stem response audiometry.

An advantage of cortical electric response audiometry is that in measuring the most central responses the entire auditory mechanism is tested. Responses can thus be best equated with clinical hearing. This is particularly important when there is a question of a central disturbance.

A major disadvantage of cortical electric response audiometry is that the potentials are also affected by sleep and sedation. Because of these factors, cortical electric response audiometry is more difficult to perform in a clinical setting and will not be discussed further.

ELECTROCOCHLEOGRAPHY

Stimulation techniques

The stimulus most commonly used in electrocochleography is a wide-band click stimulus. Acoustically the click comprises a large number of frequencies which stimulate the entire cochlea. With a flat hearing loss, the click is a good predictor of audiometric threshold. With sloping hearing losses, however, one cannot predict the type of audiogram using click stimuli.

Eggermont (1976) has used tone bursts for electrocochleography. Frequency-specific tone bursts are more accurate indicators of hearing levels at different frequencies and predict the behavioral audiogram quite accurately.

Recording techniques

A standard Teflon insulated electromyographic recording needle is positioned on to the bone of the promontory after induction of anesthesia of the tympanic membrane by means of iontophoresis or topical phenol application. Responses are filtered below 30 Hz and above 3200 Hz. The computer is set to measure over a 10 ms window.

Measurable potentials

Electrocochleography is a measure of the potentials arising within the cochlea and the auditory nerve: cochlear microphonic, summating potential, and eighth nerve action potential.

Cochlear microphonic

The source of the cochlear microphonic is the hair-bearing surface of the hair cells. Its onset is immediate and it mimics the wave form of the acoustic stimulus. Because the response recorded from the promontory is diffuse and gives no definite information regarding specific populations of hair cells, most investigators do not find the cochlear microphonic clinically useful. Gibson and Beagley (1976) are an exception and have used the cochlear microphonic to aid in differentiation of cochlear from retrocochlear lesions. They find a tendency toward a reduction in microphonics in cochlear lesions, whereas in acoustic tumors the cochlear microphonic is often normal.

The eighth nerve action potential is of primary interest in electrocochleography. This can be recorded free of interfering cochlear microphonic by cancelling the microphonic by alternating the phase of the click or tone burst stimulus.

Summating potential

The summating potential also is generated by the hair cells and is a direct current shift of the baseline of the recording, which is almost always negative for all frequencies and intensity levels in man. This potential is thought to represent asymmetry in the basilar membrane movement resulting from a pressure difference between the scala tympani and the scala vestibuli during sound stimulation (Eggermont, 1976). The source of this direct current shift is also in the hair cells. As we shall see later, this potential may be a means of studying hair cells in Ménière's disease and other cochlear disorders.

Since the summating potential appears superimposed on the eighth nerve action potential, its measurement is sometimes difficult. One technique for separating the summating potential from the eighth nerve action potential is to increase the click rate. As the rate of the click is increased, the eighth nerve action potential diminishes, because the individual neurons do not have time to recover from their refractory period to again respond to the new stimulus. The summating potential is unaffected by click rate. A recording is first done at a low click rate and the response, which comprises both the summating potential and the eighth nerve action potential, is stored in the computer. A second recording is then done with a high click rate. The response obtained represents primarily the summating potential and is used as a measure of that response. The second response can then be subtracted from the first response in the computer, and the derived response will represent primarily the eighth nerve action potential devoid of the contaminating summating potential.

Compound action potential

The eighth nerve action potential is the averaged response of the discharge pattern of many auditory neurons. Cochlear dynamics which influence the shape of the compound action potential are extremely complex and beyond the scope of this discussion. The reader is referred to Eggermont's (1976) chapter on electrocochleography in the *Handbook of Sensory Physiology* for a current review of this subject.

In addition to the normal compound action potential, Portmann and Aran (1971) have described four types of electrocochleographic response in patients with sensorineural hearing impairment: dissociated, recruiting, broad and abnormal. Only the normal response will be described here.

NORMAL RESPONSE

In patients with normal hearing an action potential can be elicited to within 5–10 dB of the patient's behavioral threshold in most cases. At high intensity the potential is large, consistent, and easily recordable and reproducible. Action potentials are described by three parameters: latency, amplitude and wave form.

Latency is defined as the time interval from the onset of the click to the maximal

negative deflection in the action potential. Latency normally decreases systematically, from approximately 4 ms at threshold to 1.5 ms at high intensity. Amplitude,
on the other hand, characteristically increases in two steps. There is a gradual rise
to the level of approximately 40 to 50 dB HL, where there is a plateau, and then a
second more rapid increase in amplitude above that level.

By convention, latency and amplitude (as a percentage of maximal amplitude)
are plotted in relation to stimulus intensity. The maximal amplitude and representative wave forms are plotted on the recording (*Figure 9.2*).

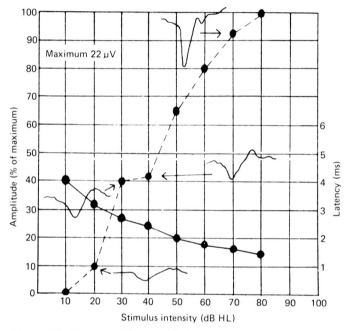

Figure 9.2 Electrocochleographic input–output function graph. Amplitude (●----●) as the
percentage of maximal amplitude and latency (●——●) are plotted against intensity of
stimulus. Representative wave forms are also shown

Clinical applications of electrocochleography

There are three clinical uses for electrocochleography: threshold testing, the study
of Ménière's disease and the study of acoustic neurinomas.

Threshold testing

Electrocochleography is the most accurate of the objective audiometric tests.
Thresholds to the click are an indication of the audiometric threshold in the 3000 to
4000 Hz range. Electrocochleographic threshold predicts the behavioral threshold
to within 5–10 dB at this frequency in almost all cases. As stated before, however,
one cannot predict the audiogram using clicks only.

There is a much better correlation to the subjective audiogram if tone bursts are used rather than clicks. The best correlation is seen at frequencies of 1, 2, and 4 kHz, but correlation remains excellent at 500 Hz and 8000 Hz.

The disadvantage of using electrocochleography for threshold determination is the necessity for transtympanic needle placement. At the Otologic Medical Group, Inc., we currently use auditory brain-stem response audiometry for threshold determination.

Ménière's disease

The summating potential and the compound action potential are of interest in the study of Ménière's disease.

SUMMATING POTENTIAL

Eggermont (1976) has found an increased negative summating potential during periods of hearing loss in the fluctuant hearing stage of Ménière's disease. He attributes this finding to either a mechanical displacement of the basilar membrane (which causes non-linearities in its movement as a result of the presumed endolymphatic hydrops) or a metabolic disturbance resulting in a larger endo-lymphatic potential. As fixed hearing loss develops, the summating potential decreases. This indicates a loss of hair cells. Measurement of the summating potential may therefore be an indication of reversibility of the hearing impairment in Ménière's disease.

COMPOUND ACTION POTENTIAL

Compound action potentials in Ménière's disease are generally of the broad type, most likely because of the contribution of a large negative summating potential.

In approximately 50% of the patients with Ménière's disease whom we studied, a distinctive type of eighth nerve action potential was found, characterized by a tendency to form multiple negative responses (Brackmann and Selters, 1976). We have not seen this type of response in other forms of sensorineural hearing loss, and this may be a means of distinguishing endolymphatic hydrops.

Acoustic neurinomas

The potential of most interest in acoustic neuroma study is the compound action potential. Gibson and Beagley (1976) have also studied the cochlear microphonic, as previously mentioned. The compound action potential in acoustic neuromas is much broader than the normal potential. In our study of 50 patients with acoustic neuromas by electrocochleography, we found an abnormal action potential in 85% (Brackmann and Selters, 1976).

As we shall see later in this presentation, brain-stem audiometry is a more accurate predictor of acoustic tumors, and we use it exclusively for this problem at the present time.

Future applications of electrocochleography

Because of the necessity of penetrating the tympanic membrane for electrocochleography, auditory brain-stem response audiometry has replaced it in most clinics. Threshold testing is nearly as accurate with auditory brain-stem response audiometry as with electrocochleography Auditory brain-stem response audiometry is a more accurate predictor of retrocochlear pathology than is electrocochleography.

The future of electrocochleography lies in the study of cochlear and eighth nerve physiology and pathophysiology. Changes in cochlear microphonics and summating potentials are an indication of hair-cell disease. As outlined above, study of the summating potential and compound action potential are means of assessing the state of the end-organ in Ménière's disease.

Moffat (1977) has reported changes in these potentials during glycerol dehydration in patients with Ménière's disease. Gibson, Ramsden and Moffat (1977) have also demonstrated changes in these potentials with the administration of intravenous vasodilators. Electrocochleography is therefore a powerful new tool in the study of cochlear disease which will have great future application.

The disadvantage of electrocochleography is the necessity for transtympanic placement of the needle electrode. Because of this, surface recording techniques have become much more popular in the United States.

AUDITORY BRAIN-STEM RESPONSE AUDIOMETRY

Stimulation techniques

As in electrocochleography, the stimulus most commonly used for auditory brain-stem response audiometry is a wide-band click stimulus. This stimulus presents the same limitations in brain-stem audiometry as in electrocochleography in that the entire cochlea is stimulated, and one cannot predict the audiogram except in cases of flat hearing impairment.

The majority of sensorineural losses are sloping, with the loss greater in the higher frequencies. Errors might therefore occur in predicting a more severe loss than is actually present because of preservation of low tone hearing.

Relatively frequency-specific stimuli (tone bursts, tone pips, filtered clicks) may also be used to elicit the brain-stem responses. These stimuli give more frequency-specific information regarding the cochlea and may be used to estimate audiometric thresholds, as described later.

Recording techniques

Standard electrocochleographic disc electrodes are attached to the vertex and both mastoids of the patient to be tested. The vertex electrode is the active lead, with the mastoid on the stimulated side the reference electrode and the mastoid of the unstimulated ear the ground electrode. Band-passing of the system occurs at 30 to 3000 Hz, with an overall amplification of 100 000. A time window of 10 ms is used.

Sedation is not used in adults or in small infants, who often sleep during the procedure. Uncooperative children are sedated as follows: 1 ml/11.3 kg (25 lb) intramuscularly of a combination of Demerol 25 mg, promethazine (Phenergan) 6.25 mg, and Thorazine 6.25 mg per 1 ml. A maximum of 1 ml is used. Chloral hydrate 500 mg/5 ml in an oral dose of 1–2 ml/4.5 kg (10 lb) may be used in place of the injectable medication.

Normal brain-stem responses

A series of seven waves may be recorded from the scalp vertex during the first 10 ms following sound stimulation. These waves are thought to represent successive synapses in the auditory pathway, with wave V most likely representing the inferior colliculus. Of these various responses, wave V is the one that is most consistent and is used in the clinical assessment of hearing (*Figure 9.3*).

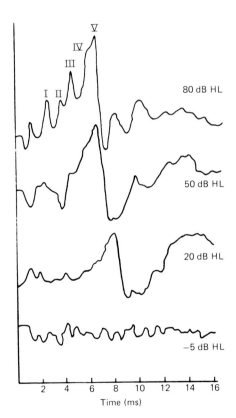

Figure 9.3 Normal brain-stem responses to a broad-band click. Latency increases as click intensity decreases

Frequency-following responses

Similar to the cochlear microphonic response, the frequency-following response follows the frequency of tonal stimulation. It is distinguished from the cochlear microphonic by its onset latency of about 6 ms. This has led to the general consensus that its origin is in the region of the inferior colliculus. Some researchers are still investigating whether the frequency-following response could possibly be a repeated wave V of the transient brain-stem response.

Recently Davis and Hirsh (1976, 1979), Suzuki and Horiuchi (1977) and Suzuki, Hirai and Horiuchi (1977) have described another response at around 10 ms after stimulus onset. Davis and Hirsh have labeled this the SN-10 response and believe that the generator is the primary auditory cortex.

The first appearance and the latency of wave V are the measures most used in brain-stem audiometry. Wave V latency is dependent upon stimulus intensity: as the intensity of the stimulus is increased, there is a systematic shortening of the latency, from about 8.5 ms at threshold to 5.5 ms at 60 dB hearing level.

Clinical applications of auditory brain-stem response audiometry

There are three major clinical uses of brain-stem audiometry: (1) threshold testing of infants, young children, and malingerers; (2) diagnosis of acoustic neurinomas; and (3) diagnosis of brain-stem lesions.

Threshold testing

Brain-stem audiometry is used in all cases in which standard behavioral audiometric techniques fail. This technique allows identification of hearing impairment in infancy so that rehabilitation can be started. As described above, wide-band click stimuli stimulate the entire cochlea, and one cannot predict the audiogram except in cases of flat hearing impairment. Despite this deficiency, the technique is valuable for early identification of hearing loss. If an error is made, it is usually in predicting a greater hearing loss than is actually present. In either case, early rehabilitation is begun.

Kodera *et al.* (1977) have shown good correlation between the behavioral audiogram and brain-stem audiometry using tone burst stimuli. As with electrocochleography, the correlations are better for the high frequencies than the lower ones. Use of these stimuli predicts the pure tone audiogram more accurately than use of broad-band click stimuli. This technique, however, is still not able to predict low-frequency hearing accurately.

Some studies have shown good correlation of the frequency-following responses to low-frequency hearing thresholds. The disadvantage of the use of this response is that its amplitude is very small and that it is difficult to separate artifact from the response. Some researchers have questioned the area of the cochlea from which this response is initiated at moderate to high levels of stimulation. Thus, even though this response shows promise of aiding in the assessment of low-frequency hearing, many questions remain unanswered regarding its clinical applicability.

Recently we have applied a technique involving the use of high-pass noise masking which can reasonably reconstruct the pure-tone audiogram. This technique was first introduced in animal work by Teas, Eldredge and Davis (1962) and later applied to electrocochleography by Elberling (1974). In this technique the brain-stem response to the broad-band click is first recorded. Successive regions of the cochlea are then masked by high-pass masking noise. Computer manipulation of the data allows measurement of the derived response from different areas of the cochlea from which pure-tones thresholds are estimated. A good approximation of the pure-tone audiogram can be made with this technique.

The disadvantages of this technique are the time required to complete the test and the sophisticated equipment necessary. Research on methods to simplify the test is currently being conducted.

USE OF A COMBINATION OF TECHNIQUES

Davis and Hirsh (1979) have proposed that a combination of techniques be used to approximate the pure-tone audiogram. They use auditory brain-stem responses to 2 and 4 kHz tone pips to estimate the audiogram at those frequencies. The later SN-10 response to 1 and 0.5 kHz tone pips is used to estimate the hearing at those frequencies. Moushegian, Allen and Stillman (1978) have proposed that the auditory brain-stem responses be used to assess the more basal portions of the cochlea and the frequency following response to assess the apical region.

CURRENT STATUS OF THRESHOLD TESTING

At the present time, we are using broad-band click stimulation to elicit the brain-stem responses. From this we estimate the hearing in the 3 to 4 kHz region of the cochlea. We estimate the low-frequency hearing with the use of impedance audiometry. The presence of an acoustic reflex to a low-frequency stimulus indicates preservation of hearing in the lower frequencies. This finding together with an absent auditory brain-stem response to high-frequency click stimulation would indicate a sloping type high-frequency hearing loss and would be an indication for caution in fitting of a hearing aid. In such a case we might well prescribe a low-gain hearing aid with high-frequency emphasis.

On the other hand, the absence of an acoustic reflex to a low-frequency stimulus combined with an absent brain-stem response to a high-intensity click implies a profound hearing impairment and indicates the need for a high-gain hearing aid.

The use of the frequency-following response, the SN-10 response and the high-pass masking technique require further study and clinical verification. Some combination of these techniques gives promise of accurate prediction of the pure-tone audiogram with objective measuring techniques.

Acoustic neurinoma diagnosis

Auditory brain-stem response audiometry has proved to be the best audiometric test for acoustic tumor detection (Selters and Brackmann, 1977). The success of

ABR depends upon the fact that acoustic tumors stretch or compress the auditory nerve, producing a delay in the response latency, which ABR can detect. This delay may occur in an ear with normal hearing. Conversely, cochlear lesions have little effect on the brain-stem response latencies for high-intensity stimuli until the hearing loss becomes rather severe.

There are several techniques in which the latency of wave V is used for detection of a retrocochlear lesion. The first is to measure the absolute latency of the wave and compare it to normals. The normal latency for wave V is between 5 and 5.7 ms. Because of this rather large variability among normal patients, we have not found the measure of the absolute latency of wave V to be very useful in acoustic neurinoma diagnosis. Another approach has been to measure the interval between the first and fifth waves. This so-called measure of central conduction time has the advantage of removing the error which occurs when there is a high-frequency sensorineural hearing impairment producing a cochlear delay, as described below. Prolongation of the wave I–V interval should reflect only the delay of propagation of the nerve impulse along the auditory nerve secondary to tumor compression.

The difficulty with the use of this technique is that patients with either sensory hearing loss or an acoustic tumor often do not have a recordable wave I. Thus, this technique cannot be used. Coates (1978) has increased his ability to use this method by making simultaneous recordings with an ear canal electrode and scalp electrodes. The ear canal electrode more frequently detects the first wave, while the surface electrodes are used to record the fifth wave. This procedure, however, requires the placement of an ear canal electrode and also necessitates equipment which is capable of simultaneous recording.

Another difficulty in using central conduction time as the only measure of a retrocochlear lesion is that a tumor may cause delay in wave I; wave I–V latency would be normal with all of the waves delayed.

The technique which we use for acoustic tumor detection is to compare the patient's non-suspect ear with the ear with the suspected acoustic tumor. With this technique, the patient acts as his own control to reduce the variability seen between normal patients.

INTERAURAL LATENCY DIFFERENCES IN PATIENTS WITH NORMAL HEARING

Brain-stem responses to an 83 dB HL broad-band click are recorded. The non-test ear is masked by 78 dB white noise. The responses are studied for the detection and latency of wave V, which is the largest and most recordable of the peaks. The latency between the two ears (IT_5) is compared. In studying a group of normal patients, we found a difference of no more than 0.2 ms between the wave V latencies for the two ears.

INTERAURAL LATENCY DIFFERENCES IN PATIENTS WITH UNILATERAL HEARING LOSS

Non-tumor cases

Patients with hearing impairment greater than 75 dB at either 2 or 4 kHz are excluded because they do not give reliable brain-stem responses. When the hearing loss is less than 55 dB at 4 kHz, there is an insignificant effect on the wave V latency. As the hearing loss at 4 kHz increases above 50 dB, wave V latency gradually increases at the rate of about 0.1 ms per 10 dB, and it is necessary to introduce a correction factor in order to decrease the number of false positive responses.

The correction factor was determined which would eliminate the majority of the false positive responses without creating any false negatives (tumors missed), which is a much more serious error. A correction factor of 0.1 ms is subtracted for a 4 kHz pure-tone hearing loss of 55 or 60 dB, and 0.2 ms is subtracted for hearing loss of 65 or 70 dB. The data are recorded as illustrated in *Figure 9.4*.

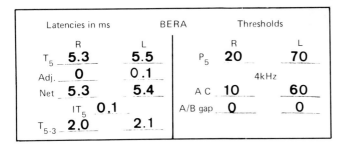

Figure 9.4 Examples of data recording from three different patients. (*Top*) Patient with normal hearing. (*Center*) Patient with an acoustic tumor. Despite correction for the high-frequency hearing loss, there is an interaural latency difference of 0.5 ms. The prolonged T_{5-3} interval indicates a large tumor. (*Bottom*) Patient with sensory hearing loss. Despite the same pure tone hearing level at 4 kHz as in the patient with the tumor, the interaural latency difference is only 0.1 ms. T_5 = latency of wave V; Adj. = correction of high-frequency hearing loss; IT_5 = interaural latency difference; T_{5-3} = latency from wave III to wave V; P_5 = detection threshold for wave V; AC = 4 kHz pure tone air conduction level; A/B gap = air–bone gap

Tumor cases

One half of patients with acoustic neurinomas have no detectable wave V, regardless of the degree of hearing impairment. We consider this indicative of an acoustic neurinoma.

Of 150 tumor patients, 96% have shown an adjusted interaural difference (IT_5) of more than 0.2 ms. Comparing ABR with the other standard neuro-otological tests, we find that ABR is the most accurate of these tests and also has the lowest false positive rate (*Table 9.2*). Brain-stem audiometry has therefore become an important part of our evaluation of acoustic tumor suspects.

Table 9.2 Failure rate of four screening tests, expressed as a percentage of the number of tests performed

	ABR	*X-ray*	*ENG*	*ART*
False negative (tumor missed)	4%	11%	23%	30%
False positive (false alarm)	8%	27%	28%	28%

ABR = auditory brain-stem audiometry;
ENG = electronystagmography; ART = acoustic reflex test.

PREDICTION OF TUMOR SIZE

Large acoustic tumors press against the brain stem. If significant pressure is exerted on the auditory tracts in the brain stem, abnormalities in the brain-stem response are detectable when testing the opposite (non-tumor) ear. This effect is best detected by measuring the interval between the third and fifth waves. Normally this interval, T_{5-3}, will be 1.9 ± 0.1 ms. A T_{5-3} of 2.1 to 2.8 ms has been found in 71% of 55 patients having tumors larger than 3 cm. Thus, brain-stem audiometry may not only predict the presence of an acoustic tumor, but also the general size of the tumor.

CONDUCTIVE HEARING LOSSES

One word of caution is in order. Conductive hearing impairments will produce latency shifts that mimic an acoustic tumor. Standard audiometric tests to rule out conductive losses should first be performed.

CURRENT USE OF ABR IN THE NEURO-OTOLOGICAL EVALUATION

Our routine evaluation of a tumor suspect includes petrous pyramid X-rays, electronystagmography (ENG), and an acoustic reflex text (ART). If the X-rays show definite enlargement of the internal auditory canal on the suspect side, a contrast study is obtained, usually computerized tomography (with air contrast if necessary), followed by a small-dose polytome Pantopaque study if the diagnosis remains in doubt after computerized tomography.

If the findings on X-ray are not definite, but the ENG or acoustic reflex test suggests a tumor, we obtain ABR. If that is positive, the contrast studies (as described above) are performed.

Recently we have used ABR as a primary screening test more often. In some cases the ENG and acoustic reflex test have been omitted because of ABR. ABR is a significant addition to the acoustic tumor detection test battery, which is being used with increasing frequency.

Non-acoustic cerebellopontine angle tumors

Twenty-eight patients with cerebellopontine angle tumors, not acoustic tumors, have been studied with brain-stem audiometry (*Table 9.3*). Brain-stem audiometry has identified the tumor in cases where there has been pressure on the cochlear nerve. Because some non-acoustic lesions of the angle do not produce pressure on the cochlear nerve, the detection rate for these tumors is not as good as for acoustic neurinomas.

Table 9.3 Detection rate for non-acoustic cerebellopontine angle tumors (28 patients)

Wave V – absent or delayed	75%
Wave V – normal in:	25%
3 of 10 meningiomas	
1 of 5 cholesteatomas	
2 of 4 facial nerve neurinomas	
arachnoid cyst	

Brain-stem lesions

Brain-stem audiometry is of distinct value in the diagnosis and localization of brain-stem lesions. Intra-axial pontine masses which impinge upon the auditory tracts produce loss of brain-stem responses. The level of the mass can be predicted on the basis of the presence or absence of succeeding brain-stem responses (Starr and Achor, 1975). Absence of brain-stem responses is an early indication of multiple sclerosis in a large percentage of those patients (Stockard, Stockard and Sharbrough, 1977). Lesions in the auditory tract produce desynchronization of the responses, which makes them non-detectable despite the presence of normal pure-tone and speech audiometry in many cases.

CONCLUSIONS

Electric response audiometry is an exciting new development with broad implications in the fields of otology, audiology and neurology. At the present time it is the best objective audiometric test for predicting hearing thresholds in infants and uncooperative patients.

Electrocochleography offers a means for the study of the function of the inner ear and for the differentiation of types of sensorineural hearing impairment. Auditory brain-stem response audiometry is a valuable addition to the audiological test battery for the diagnosis of acoustic tumors. It also offers a means of studying brain-stem function in a variety of neurological disorders.

Acknowledgement

This work was sponsored by a grant from the House Ear Institute, an affiliate of the University of Southern California School of Medicine, Los Angeles.

References

Brackmann, D. E. and Selters, W. A. (1976) Electrocochleography in Ménière's disease and acoustic neuromas. In *Electrocochleography*, edited by R. J. Ruben, C. Elberling and G. Salomon, pp. 315–329. Baltimore: University Park Press

Coates, A. C. (1978) Human auditory nerve action potential and brain stem evoked response latency-intensity functions in detection of cochlear and retrocochlear pathology. *Archives of Otolaryngology*, **104**, 809–817

Davis, H. and Hirsh, S. K. (1976) The audiometric utility of brain stem responses to low-freqency sounds. *Audiology*, **15**, 181–195

Davis, H. and Hirsh, S. K. (1979) A slow brain stem response for low-frequency audiometry. *Audiology*, **18**, 445–461

Don, M., Eggermont, J. J. and Brackmann, D. E. (1979) Reconstructing the audiogram using brain stem responses and high-pass noise masking. *Annals of Otology, Rhinology and Laryngology*, **88** (Suppl. 57), May–June, 1–20

Eggermont, J. J. (1976) Electrocochleography. In *Auditory System (Part 3): Clinical and Special Topics*, edited by W. D. Keidel and W. D. Neff. *Handbook of Sensory Physiology*, **5**. Berlin: Springer Verlag

Elberling, C. (1974) Action potentials along the cochlear partition recorded from the ear canal in man. *Scandinavian Audiology*, **3**, 13–19

Gibson, W. P. R. and Beagley, H. A. (1976) Transtympanic electrocochleography in the investigation of the retrolabyrinthine disorders. *Revue de Laryngologie, Otologie, Rhinologie*, **97**, 507–516

Gibson, W. P. R., Ramsden, R. T. and Moffat, D. A. (1977) The immediate effects of naftidrofuryl on the human electrocochleogram in Ménière's disorder – preliminary findings. *Journal of Laryngology and Otology*, **91**, 679–696

Kodera, K., Yamane, H., Yamada, O. and Suzuki, J.-I. (1977) Brain stem response audiometry at speech frequencies. *Audiology*, **16**, 469–479

Moffat, D. A. (1977) Transtympanic electrocochleography during glycerol dehydration. (Paper read at Fifth Symposium of International ERA Study Group, Jerusalem, 1977)

Moushegian, G., Allen, R. L. and Stillman, R. D. (1978) Evaluation of frequency-following potentials in man: masking and clinical studies. *EEG and Clinical Neurophysiology*, **45**, 711–818

Portmann, M. and Aran, J. M. (1971) Electrocochleography. *Laryngoscope*, **81**, 899–910

Selters, W. A. and Brackmann, D. E. (1977) Acoustic tumor detection with brain stem electric response audiometry. *Archives of Otolaryngology*, **103**, 181–187

Starr, A. and Achor, J. (1975) Auditory brain stem responses in neurological disease. *Archives of Neurology*, **32**, 761–868

Stockard, J. J., Stockard, J. E. and Sharbrough, F. W. (1977) Detection and localization of occult lesions with brain stem auditory responses. *Mayo Clinic Proceedings*, **52**, 761–869

Suzuki, T., Hirai, Y. and Horiuchi, K. (1977) Auditory brain stem responses to pure tone stimuli. *Scandinavian Audiology*, **6**, 51–56

Suzuki, T. and Horiuchi, K. (1977) Effect of high-pass filter on auditory brain stem responses to tone pips. *Scandinavian Audiology*, **6**, 123–126

Teas, D. C., Eldredge, D. H. and Davis, H. (1962) Cochlear responses to acoustic transients: an interpretation of whole-nerve action potentials. *Journal of the Acoustical Society of America*, **34**, 1483–1489

10
Non-organic hearing loss

R. Ross A. Coles

Non-organic hearing loss (NOHL) is quite common in all forms of otological and audiological practice, but its incidence therein varies enormously. This depends on the kind of practice and the extent to which both medical and non-medical staff are alert to it and take positive measures to detect it. Indeed, a department complacent in this respect may have an apparent incidence of NOHL that is close to zero (Doerfler, 1951).

I have had a particular interest in this subject due to my medical audiological practice in the Royal Navy and later in an audiological diagnostic reference centre and in medicolegal work. Much of the data presented in this chapter relates to analysis of 70 cases of NOHL seen at Southampton up to 1970, increasing to 264 cases up to 1977, and to electric response audiometry tests carried out in 118 medicolegal cases in Nottingham over the last 2 years.

In the past, NOHL has been referred to as either psychogenic or hysterical deafness, or feigned or simulated deafness (malingering). In reality, these are but the extremes of a continuum and not appropriate to the majority of cases in that continuum. The more embracing term 'non-organic hearing loss', which refers to any measured hearing loss that does not have a basis in organic pathology, is much better. The hearing loss may or may not be accompanied by subjective symptoms of deafness or hearing difficulty compatible with the measured loss. Thus, NOHL is essentially a descriptive term for a particular audiometric finding rather than a particular abnormal condition in its own right. There are advantages in adhering to the audiometric definition of NOHL, since it is the apparent hearing loss which is the presenting feature of the condition, and that which may cause diagnostic error.

I therefore define NOHL as 'any substantial difference between an apparent hearing level and the true hearing level'. 'Substantial' in this context means 20 dB or more and the 'apparent' hearing level is that measured in a person who is old enough and apparently intelligent and fit enough to perform satisfactorily in audiometry and who seems to have done so. In this definition, hearing loss due to instrument failure is excluded.

CLASSIFICATION

The psychogenic form of NOHL is rarely seen. On the other hand, there do seem to be a number of persons who have simply lost confidence in their ability to hear, so that they fail to respond to any pure-tone or speech signals below a certain elevated level (possibly their comfortable listening level). Quite often, during the investigation their confidence gradually returns with increasing ease of hearing of speech in conversation, especially when not in a formal test environment.

The other extreme, that of deliberate feigning or exaggeration without any psychogenic overlay, is also uncommon. Coles and Priede (1971) have therefore proposed a classification which includes two additional categories: mixed (psychogenic and feigned) and artefactual. This is described below.

Purely psychogenic NOHL

To diagnose this with certainty, rather strict criteria have to be applied (Goldstein, 1967), which effectively make it an extremely rare form of NOHL. I may have seen three cases, but am not sure.

Purely feigned NOHL

Like Goldstein, we have observed a psychogenic element in most malingerers. To put a case of NOHL into this category therefore becomes a question of how small that element must be. That in turn must depend on the purpose for which categorization of aetiology of NOHL is required.

Mixed NOHL

This comprises the vast majority of cases. It has five subcategories according to the type of psychogenic element.

(1) Anxiety concerning hearing ability for work. Associated with the simulation or exaggeration there is an underlying anxiety or loss of confidence concerning hearing. This is particularly common where hearing is of prime importance to the job, e.g. in telephonists or radio operators. Usually there has been some stressful experience, such as being accused of inattentiveness. In some cases there is also a real disorder of hearing.
(2) Anxiety concerning ears, hearing or tinnitus. There may be fear of progression of the disorder, and exaggeration becomes a means of gaining greater attention. Children may use it to attract parental attention or avoid stresses at school. In adults, it sometimes occurs when a hearing conservation programme is first instituted, especially in those who have experienced prominent tinnitus or dullness of hearing following noise exposure.

(3) Anxiety not related to the ears or hearing.
(4) Psychopathic personality and delinquency.
(5) Psychosis.

Artefactual NOHL

The subcategories which comprise this classification are the following. As already stated, incorrect audiograms due to instrument failure have been excluded.

(1) Misunderstanding of audiometric task. Probably the most common cause of error in audiometry is the failure to give adequate instructions or to make certain that the patient understands what he has to do. Its avoidance is a matter of proper training and supervision.
(2) Inattention at audiometry. This is frequently the cause of poor results in children, the elderly and the mentally subnormal. Its recognition is a matter of observation and experience.
(3) Meatus occlusion by the audiometer earphone. This can happen in three kinds of patients: the chubby child, the elderly where the meatal skin has lost its elasticity, and the adult with a deformed pinna, e.g. a 'cauliflower ear' as a sequel to a perichondrial haematoma. The incidence of such inadvertent meatus closure may be as high as 0.5% in a typical otological practice.

   The audiometric effect is of a mild high-tone hearing loss like the attenuation effect of an ear-plug, about 10 dB at low frequencies, rising to 30 or 40 dB at high frequencies around 4000 Hz, and sometimes less at 8000 Hz. The artefact is limited to the air conduction tests. Such cases are identified by disagreement between an unexpected high-frequency conductive hearing loss and the results of tuning fork tests or the presence of acoustic reflexes. If such an artefact is suspected, the hearing should be measured with a hollowed-out bung in the ear, e.g. a temporary hearing aid insert or an impedance meter probe tip, which holds the meatus open under the earphone (Coles, 1967).

INCIDENCE

The incidence of NOHL in a particular otological or audiological clinic depends obviously on the kind of cases referred to it. In my experience the majority of children who appear to have developed sensorineural hearing loss between the ages of 6 and 16 years have no demonstrable organic pathology. Shortcomings in the initial testing elsewhere often lead to a high rate of referral of these children for further investigation of 'unexpected deafness'.

   Amongst the author's medicolegal cases claiming chronic noise-induced hearing loss, the incidence of NOHL was about 35%; but this reflects the fact that many of them were referred precisely because of uncertainty about the degree or nature of their deafness. In an unselected group of compensation claimants, Alberti, Morgan and Le Blanc (1974) reported a NOHL incidence of 20%, but a disturbingly high proportion of otologists seemed to be very poor at picking up such cases (Alberti, 1981a). The incidence of NOHL is higher still in cases of unilateral hearing loss allegedly due to acute acoustic trauma (e.g. blast injury) or head injury, perhaps because of the more obvious litigational possibilities, but often linked to a sense of grievance and the patient's genuine belief that he is deaf or hard-of-hearing in one ear.

On the other hand, in the general audiological case load of adults referred to the author's clinic at Southampton for specialist auditory investigations, the incidence of NOHL has only been about 1%. Even this may be an inflated figure and the incidence in the general otology clinic population may be lower still, although Doerfler (1951) found it to vary between 0 and over 5% in a survey of 30 leading audiology centres in the USA whose cases were mostly referred by otologists.

DETECTION

Detection of NOHL depends on observation of the patient's behaviour, certain suggestive features in clinical and audiometric presentation, a whole range of anomalous results in ordinary audiometric tests (indicator tests), and the results of tests specifically designed or used to detect NOHL (proof tests). It is also greatly assisted by a heightened vigilance for these signs in cases where there may be some motivation towards NOHL; this often becomes apparent when taking the history, both in adults and in children.

Observation of the patient

Attitude

One might expect patients with NOHL to be somewhat evasive, but this is uncommon. Indeed, the expression '*la belle indifference*' would quite often seem to apply, even though the subsequently discovered NOHL is rarely of the hysterical type. On the other hand, there are NOHL patients who do exaggerate certain aspects of their disorder, either in their history, when it is difficult to detect the exaggeration, or in their general demeanour. Presumably in an attempt to impress, they are apt – in a rather forced way – to put their supposedly better ear forward, to cup their hand to their ear, or to make exaggerated use of their hearing aid. Particularly suspicious is the patient who manages reasonably well during the history taking but then volunteers or admits to being highly dependent on lip-reading; he may also watch your lips with avid concentration or deny hearing anything when he cannot see them. Others may avoid watching your face; such behaviour in a patient who is allegedly deaf or works in high levels of noise is most suspicious.

Hearing ability

It is good practice generally, and particularly helpful for the detection of NOHL, to note the patient's ability to hear during history taking and especially at other, less formal, times. The audiological staff should be instructed to do likewise and report any discrepancies. Such 'tests' can be contrived; for example, while examining the ear it is possible to ask questions in various levels of voice, e.g. if the aural speculum is quite comfortable. Examination for spontaneous nystagmus under Frenzel glasses gives another useful opportunity, as does the fitting of earphones or an impedance probe by the technician. Visual and auditory observation of patients during electric response audiometry (ERA) may also be revealing: one patient was even heard to softly count the tone pips which were being presented to him at a level which he totally denied hearing.

The hearing aid should always be inspected, preferably without the patient taking it off himself, in order to see at what volume it is set. This allows an estimate of how much amplification the patient is using in order to hear the examiner. Also check that the hearing aid is actually turned on, the function selector is in the correct 'M' position, and that it is functioning. Some NOHL patients seem to hear quite well when in fact they are wearing an aid with no battery or a run-down battery, or suffering from a blocked acoustic tube, or some other major malfunction.

Voice

The sound and level of voice should be noted, since occasionally a patient claiming severe hearing loss of long standing may have a normal-sounding voice and normal voice level. This discrepancy should give rise to suspicion of NOHL.

Eyes

Discrepancies in or abnormalities of lip-reading behaviour have already been mentioned.

Presentation

Clinical presentation

NOHL is widespread. Our data suggest that it is more common in girls than in boys. Medicolegal and occupational assessments of the effects of noise concern chiefly male employees. Otherwise the adult incidence is approximately equal (*Table 10.1*).

It has sometimes been said that the higher incidence of NOHL in girls is related to stresses associated with the menarche. This seems unlikely from our own data (*Figure 10.1*), which show somewhat similar peaks in ages of maximum incidence of NOHL for boys and girls. A possible explanation may be the stresses associated with examinations at school. Much of the case material was collected at a time when the 'eleven-plus' examination for secondary school selection prevailed.

Adult cases are found in all social and occupational groups, but our clinical impression is that they are frequently in rather unintelligent people. Indeed, the

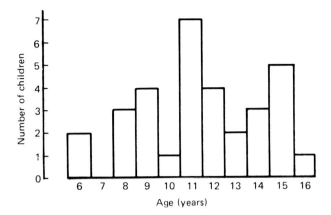

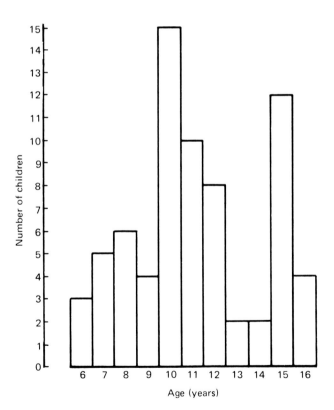

Figure 10.1 Age distribution of NOHL in 32 male (*top*) and 71 female children (median, upper and lower quartile ages are: 11.9, 9.8 and 14.3 years, male; 11.3, 9.1 and 14.2 years, female). (Note: children under 6 were excluded as NOHL cases as they may have been too young for reliable audiometry; over 16s are classified as adults)

Table 10.1 Sex distribution of NOHL in 264 cases (1966–77 sample), and breakdown of adult cases

	Male	Female	Total
Children (6–16 years)	32	71	103
Adults	134	27	161
Armed Services	71	–	
Medicolegal (occupational deafness)	28	–	
Head trauma	13	5	
Residual ('pure' NOHL)	22	22	

extreme naïvety of the exaggerations of some patients has caused astonishment and even irritation in the audiological staff concerned.

NOHL can appear in both ears (symmetrically or asymmetrically) or in just one ear, the latter most commonly as a result of head or acoustic trauma. It can be pure NOHL or a non-organic overlay. Our cases include approximately equal proportions of pure non-organic disorder and non-organic overlay, the pure ones being more common in children and the overlay ones more common in occupational deafness claimants. The degree of apparent deafness is moderate, that is, the patient hears a voice if it is quite loud but not otherwise. This equates to about 60–80 dB in the middle audiometric frequencies (500–2000 Hz). Presumably this is related to experience of common speech levels, allowing the patient to complain consistently of difficulties with anything which is not easy to hear while not having to feign severe deafness. In our analysis of the 264 cases of non-organic hearing loss seen up to 1977, total bilateral NOHL was seen in only 12 patients (5%), but a further 15 showed total unilateral NOHL.

Audiometric presentation

Patients with NOHL and underlying noise-induced hearing loss usually do not know that the degree of hearing loss should be different at different frequencies. They therefore set up approximately the same responding criterion, in terms of loudness, at each test frequency. However, in underlying noise-induced hearing loss cases the frequency range in which the cochlea has been most damaged will display recruitment of loudness, and hence the patient's audiometric responses will approximate to an equal loudness contour. The greater the exaggeration, the less any true noise-induced dip in the audiogram will show. This is well illustrated by serial audiometry, as shown in *Figure 10.2*. This young seaman had suffered prominent temporary hearing loss and tinnitus through gunblast and then became increasingly anxious about his hearing ability. Serial audiograms showed progressive deterioration, quite unlike the usual pattern of gradual recovery from an acoustic trauma, the configuration of the audiogram flattening out as the severity of

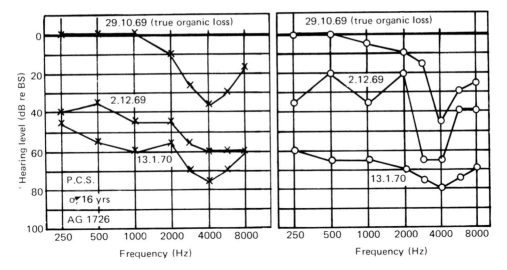

Figure 10.2 Development of non-organic overlay in a case of acute acoustic trauma (courtesy of the Editor and Publishers, *Proceedings of the Royal Society of Medicine*, Coles and Priede, 1971)

the apparent hearing loss increased. Objective tests carried out 2½ months after the original audiogram showed that the true hearing loss had not changed.

Analysis of the first 70 cases in this series led us to conclude that 'the non-organic element of the hearing loss was almost exclusively of perceptive type although it could be superimposed on an organic loss of conductive type; this is to be expected because where deafness is being feigned it is likely to apply to sounds delivered by both air conduction and bone conduction' (Coles and Priede, 1971). This was not confirmed in our 1977 analysis; in fact, we found it to be quite common for the bone conduction thresholds to be 20–40 dB more acute than the air conduction ones.

Indicators in general audiometric tests

Pure-tone audiometry (PTA)

VARIABILITY OF RESPONSE

Most patients give fairly repeatable responses within tests, except immediately around the threshold, where by definition there is a transition from heard to not heard. Some patients show differences of 10 dB or more between ascending and descending approaches to threshold, anticipating stimuli in the descending mode and failing to respond to sounds in the ascending mode until well above threshold. The majority of these and other forms of variation are not due to NOHL. But non-organic cases sometimes give 20–30 dB more acute thresholds in the ascending mode than in the descending (Harris, 1958; Kerr, Gillespie and Easton, 1975).

Neither excessive within-test nor between-test variability can be regarded as axiomatic of NOHL; indeed, some patients give remarkably consistent audiometric performances. In our 1977 analysis, 48% of the adult NOHL cases and 31% of the children gave precise responses, with differences between one pure-tone audiogram and another not exceeding 15 dB at more than one frequency.

NATURE OF RESPONSE
Whenever the test facility permits, the patient should be in the same room as the tester and indicate his responses by raising his finger for the duration of the signal. Much can be learned about the patient by observing his finger movements and general demeanour during audiometry. The delayed response of the 'malingafinger' (Green, 1978) or response button is often seen in NOHL.

COMPARISON WITH OBSERVED AUDITORY DISABILITY
It is helpful if the clinician routinely assesses the patient's hearing ability at interview, e.g., in terms of very slight, slight, moderate, moderate-to-severe, severe or profound hardness of hearing. However, since these qualititative assessments will differ considerably from one clinician to another, it is necessary to calibrate one's initial judgement against subsequent measurements. In practice, this is the most important single detector of NOHL. Systematically applied and calibrated clinical judgement could save large sums of money in cases coming up for compensation assessment, particularly within statutory schemes, where the time for audiological investigation is often very limited.

AIR CONDUCTION 'SHADOW TESTS'
Interaural attenuation data have recently been reviewed, and extended, by Smith and Markides (1981). Interaural attenuation values are to some extent frequency-dependent, but an overall figure for the maximum attenuation would seem to be 85 dB at any one frequency. Averaged across 250, 500, 1000, 2000 and 4000 Hz, Coles and Priede (1970) reported a mean value of 63 dB, with a range of 51–70 dB (Coles, unpublished observation). This means that an apparent not-masked difference between the two ears exceeding 85 dB at an individual frequency or 70 dB averaged over a range of frequencies, is unlikely to be organic in origin, i.e. the shadow is not where it should be. In our 1977 analysis of NOHL cases, left/right (L/R) threshold differences of 70 dB or more at three or more frequencies were found in only 6%. But, since the 'test' requires no more than routine threshold audiometry without use of masking, it yields a very worthwhile dividend.

BONE CONDUCTION 'SHADOW TESTS'
Although, for definition of need for masking, it is common audiological practice to regard the bone conduction (b-c) transcranial transmission loss as being zero, Snyder (1973) has shown it to have mean values of 8 to 13 dB from 250 to 4000 Hz, ranging from −15 to +20 dB at 250 Hz to −5 to +40 dB at 4000 Hz. For purposes of defining the b-c shadow test, we have taken the maximum organic b-c transmission loss averaged across three or more frequencies to be less than 15 dB.

Note that our practice has always been to put the bone conductor first on the ear with the worst air-conduction (a-c) thresholds. However, unlike in a-c tests, it is quite plain which ear is being tested, and some patients are surprised, and do not respond, if the b-c signal is heard on the contralateral side. Therefore it is essential to remind the patient just before the b-c test to respond whenever he hears a tone, no matter in which ear he hears it. In our 1977 analysis of NOHL patients, 83 had unilateral or asymmetrical apparent hearing loss, and the b-c shadow test detected NOHL in 44 of them (53%). One example is shown in *Figure 10.3*. Again, this test amounts to a very inexpensive bonus.

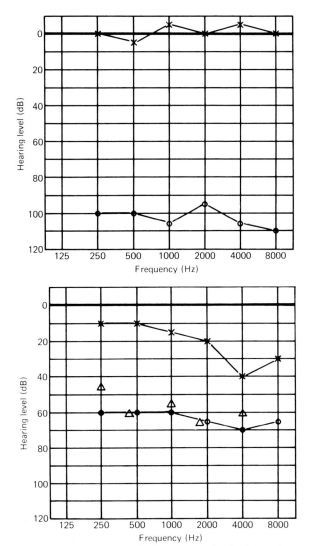

Figure 10.3 Positive 'shadow tests': (*top*) air conduction; (*bottom*) bone conduction (△ = not-masked bone-conduction; vibrator on worst a-c side; patient told to respond to any tones heard in *either* ear)

STENGER TEST

This can be done qualitatively either with tuning forks or by using a conversational or whispered voice on the 'deaf' side. However, the pure-tone audiometer version is much the best since it allows a quantitative check on the apparent difference in threshold between the two ears at any frequency of interest. If NOHL is demonstrated, the test is then extended to measure the real threshold difference between the ears. The method used in our clinic has been described by Coles and Priede in 1971, but one minor correction and some further details can now be added in the light of a later methodological study (Shammas, 1974), which showed that the true threshold difference is usually within 10 dB of (W-B), where W = lowest level (transition level) presented to the worst ear that resulted in over 50% of 'not heard' responses, and B = the constant level of tones presented to the better ear. This differs by 5 dB from the value found by Coles and Priede, who defined the transition level as 'the highest level presented to the worst ear that failed to interfere with the hearing of the good ear'.

Shammas showed that 90% of predictions of the L/R threshold differences were within ± 10 dB of the actual difference and virtually all of them within ± 15 dB. He also confirmed that the test could be carried out satisfactorily with a single-oscillator two-channel audiometer with reasonably careful manipulation of two separate signal-presentation switches.

Our data analysis of 1977 showed that the Stenger test was used in 77 cases of NOHL. It demonstrated little or no true L/R difference in 53 cases (69%) and confirmed the presence of an underlying asymmetrical hearing loss, but with a non-organic overlay, in another 10 (13%). It was not useful in 14 (18%): in 12 of these the audiometric responses were too variable for the test to be interpreted. The Stenger test failed due to diplacusis binauralis in one case and vibrotactile sensation in the other.

The Stenger check test appears to be very reliable in detecting unilateral NOHL of more than 10 dB magnitude. It takes only about one minute to perform and requires no special instructions, the patient being unaware that he is being specially checked. To perform any test efficiently requires regular practice. We therefore routinely use the check test at one frequency as part of our pure-tone threshold measurements, before any time is spent on masking and other tests, whenever any apparent L/R threshold difference reaches or exceeds 20 dB. This ensures that cases of unilateral or asymmetrical NOHL seldom pass through the clinic undetected.

Speech audiometry tests

VARIABILITY OF RESPONSE AND FOURNIER TEST TECHNIQUE

In a single ear at any particular test level, the identification scores from standardized lists of test words are usually fairly constant. For example, a difference of over 30% between lists having 30 scorable items would be unusual to the point of alerting the technician. Where NOHL is suspected it is therefore helpful to retest at one or more levels in order to check the repeatability of the response and if possible displace it. In particular, a loudness alteration technique like that advocated by Fournier in 1956 is recommended. This involves repeated lowering and raising of the test level by, for instance, 25 dB and 15 dB. When successive data points are plotted and connected by lines, many NOHL patients show a characteristic zig-zag pattern, with an ever-decreasing apparent threshold of hearing for the speech test material. In this way, NOHL patients can often be worked down towards their true thresholds. This technique can also be applied for pure-tone testing, but the simple stimuli and short intervals tend to make the procedure somewhat transparent.

In children, it is often helpful to make the speech audiometry into a competitive game. Several times we have seen an allegedly deaf child achieve a correct score to his mother's responses when the intercom, by which the mother's voice could be heard, was turned right down to levels barely audible even to the normal-hearing technician.

ANOMALOUS RESPONSES

NOHL adults are sometimes 'too clever' and give themselves away with the following forms of abnormal response: correct response to every second or third test word; all-or-none responses, i.e. no part-correct responses; always getting the first or last phoneme wrong; frequent use of alternatives, e.g. 'cat or bat', as if to impress the technician that they are trying hard; use of semantically related answers when thinking up error responses, e.g. 'left' for 'right', 'cat' for 'dog', 'boat' for 'ship'.

COMPARISON WITH PURE-TONE THRESHOLDS

If the patient is responding correctly and there is no unduly steep or peaky pure-tone audiometric configuration, there is a probability of about 90% that the speech threshold will equate to within ±10 dB of the best two of the pure-tone thresholds at 0.5, 1 and 2 kHz, after slope-factor corrections (Coles, Markides and Priede, 1973). Subsequently, Markides (1980) has shown that in children the best two of the wider frequency range 0.25, 0.5, 1, 2 and 4 kHz gives a better correlation still.

NOHL patients tend to do relatively better with speech than with pure-tone tests (Coles and Priede, 1976). In feigning cases this may be due to the greater difficulty of judging what level of speech should be responded to. In anxiety, confusion and inattention cases it is probably related to the more natural and interesting task involved in speech audiometry. Speech audiometry had been carried out in 218 of the NOHL cases included in our 1977 analysis. It indicated the true thresholds in 50%, thresholds lower than the tonal ones by 20 dB or more in 38%, thresholds consistent with the tonal ones in 11%, and worse than the tonal ones in only 1%.

Thus, skilful use of well-calibrated speech audiometry is a powerful tool for the detection of NOHL. Indeed, in many cases it reveals the true threshold also.

Acoustic impedance and reflex tests

These can help in the detection of NOHL in three ways.

RELATION TO AIR–BONE GAP

The tendency of NOHL patients to perform better in b-c than in a-c tests has already been pointed out. This often produces an apparent air–bone gap.

However, the finding of normal acoustic reflexes by ipsilateral or contralateral stimulation with the impedance probe in an ear showing an apparent air–bone gap of 10 dB or more is anomalous and highly suggestive of NOHL, or at least an artefact or error in the pure-tone audiometry. This is because in a middle ear disorder associated with a true air–bone gap of over 10 dB at several frequencies it is rare to find any acoustic reflex responses at all with the probe in the affected ear, and, if present, these are usually of abnormal quality, e.g. the inverse deflections of diphasic (on–off) type said to be highly specific for otosclerosis (Terkildsen, Osterhammel and Bretlau, 1973).

COMPARISON OF ACOUSTIC REFLEX THRESHOLD (ART) WITH HEARING THRESHOLD

Only above a hearing loss of about 55 dB does the median ART begin to rise, and then only so gradually that in individuals with hearing losses of up to 65 dB the ART can still be less than the normal average value (Priede and Coles, 1974). At the other end of the normal ART range, Anderson and Wedenberg (1968) reported 90th percentile values of 91–98 dB HL in the frequency range of 250–3000 Hz, and Priede (1973) found upper limit values in apparently normal adults to be even higher, 110 and 120 dB HL from 1000 and 4000 Hz stimuli. Thus, due to the wide range of normal values, the effects of recruitment, and the possibility of defects in other parts of the acoustic reflex arc, ART values for tonal stimuli are of little use on their own either for diagnosis or for prediction of the hearing level. Even when compared with auditory threshold values, the interpretative criteria in terms of recruitment that can be derived are distinctly limited in their scope (Priede and Coles, 1974). However, such comparisons can be helpful as indicators of the presence of NOHL.

It is almost inconceivable that an acoustic stimulus that is not audible could at the same time be 'loud' enough to initiate an acoustic reflex. Whilst the use of the acoustic reflex threshold was originally conceived as a measure of recruitment (Metz, 1952), this does not necessarily have to depend on the actual sensation of loudness, as might be inferred from the original name of the phenomenon, 'recruitment of loudness'. Indeed, Metz himself stated that in the muscle reflex 'the cerebral process is excluded'. The central component of the acoustic reflex arc is essentially a brain stem one, although Borg (1973) has shown that its innervation involves multiple polysynaptic pathways in addition to a simple reflex arc, and other studies have shown that the reflex dynamics are influenced by a number of other factors, such as eye closure (but not darkness) and distracting mental tasks (Corcoran, Cleaver and Stephens, 1980). The reflex responses are also modified, but not abolished, by sedation and sleep. Thus, although cerebral and other influences cannot be discounted, the presence or absence of acoustic reflexes is mainly determined by the function of the ear and the rest of the acoustic reflex arc, including that part within the brain stem. It is therefore possible, at least in theory, for an auditory disorder due to malfunction at cerebral level to result in severe deafness yet leave the acoustic reflexes relatively normal. Where there is any material possibility of such a disorder, great caution is needed in the interpretation of acoustic reflex measurements in terms of hearing ability.

Subject to such care, the presence of NOHL can be inferred where the ART is lower than or equal to the corresponding volunteered threshold. Where the ART is 5 or 10 dB higher than the volunteered threshold, some doubt arises due to the variability inherent in both measurements, but the data of Priede and Coles (1974) would suggest that even in cases of sensorineural hearing loss with marked degrees of recruitment, a pure-tone ART is rarely within 15 dB of the corresponding auditory threshold. Where ART and HL values are taken over several frequencies, more stringent criteria may be applied: NOHL is probably present where the ARTs average less than 10 dB higher than the corresponding auditory thresholds at two or more frequencies. Using this criterion in our 1977 analysis, we found that ART data indicated the probable presence of NOHL in 20% of those subsequently found to have it. In 15% the acoustic impedance and reflex measurements gave further information of value in that they demonstrated the presence of some middle ear disorder. In the remainder (66%) the tests were not useful except to demonstrate the absence of significant middle ear disorder. However, this analysis did not include any study of the extent to which the NOHL patients exhibited apparent air–bone gaps in the presence of normal acoustic reflexes; to judge from later experience, such study would probably have provided a further useful yield from the test.

COMPARISON OF ART FOR TONES WITH ART FOR NOISE
Niemeyer and Sesterhenn (1974) were the first to devise a means of estimating the hearing threshold from ART data by using the following equation:

$$\text{Predicted threshold} = \text{ART}_t - 2.5\,(\text{ART}_t - \text{ART}_n)$$

where the predicted threshold (dB HL) is the mean over the 0.5–4 kHz range, ART_t is the mean ART (dB HL) over the 0.5–4 kHz range, and ART_n is the ART for wide-band noise (dB relative to mean normal auditory threshold for that noise).

Their method was soon developed by Jerger *et al.* (1974) into a useful test for detection and quantification of hearing loss in children, and other predictive methods based on ART measurements have subsequently been devised (Johnsen *et al.*, 1976; Sesterhenn and Breuninger, 1977). However, Jerger, Hayes and Anthony (1978) have shown that predictive accuracy is much reduced in adults, and Hyde *et al.* (1980), after an analysis of its effectiveness in a series of 1207 patients with presumed noise-induced hearing loss, conclude that 'none of the predictions studied is adequate for medico-legal assessment and the method is probably not sufficiently accurate for clinical use in adults'.

Békésy audiometry

The use of self-recording audiometry to compare the thresholds obtained from interrupted tones with those from continuous tones has been well established in clinical practice for more than 20 years now (Jerger, 1960). It amounts to a graphical representation of auditory adaptation at threshold, or tone decay. Jerger type I patterns of response are found in conductive hearing loss. Jerger type II is found in sensory disorders and is characterized by a small amount of tone decay at the higher frequencies, the thresholds for continuous tones being up to 20 dB less acute than those for interrupted tones. Types III and IV show much greater tone decay and are found in neural disorders. Three aspects of its results can be suggestive of the presence of NOHL.

TYPE V PATTERN

Not long after the publication of Jerger's original paper it became apparent that there was another group of patients in whom the apparent thresholds for the continuous tones were more acute than those for the interrupted tones, a sort of reverse tone decay. This pattern was found in patients with NOHL and was called type V (Jerger and Herer, 1961). Our own experience is that the type V pattern is present in only about 50% of NOHL patients when the criterion is a complete separation of the interrupted tone and continuous tone traces. Incomplete type V patterns are seen, but they are sometimes also found in organic cases.

INCONSISTENCY WITH MANUAL THRESHOLDS DETERMINATION

In some NOHL cases, the Békésy threshold levels differ from those measured by normal manual audiometric methods by as much as 15 dB or more, particularly for continuous tones, the self-recorded thresholds usually being the more acute. Occasionally, the self-recorded thresholds are worse than the manual ones, and this may be associated with the difficulties which some patients apparently find in this form of audiometry.

REVERSED AND CONVERGING SWEEPS

Various other strategies have been used with self-recording audiometry in order to elicit the inconsistent responses liable to occur in NOHL. However, these require special techniques which are normally outside the scope of routine investigation, even when NOHL is suspected.

Although Békésy audiometry has much to offer in both general audiological and medicolegal investigations, there is always the need to restrict the range of tests to those which are most cost-effective. An individual's diagnostic strategy is obviously governed by many factors, but Békésy audiometry no longer holds a place in my choice of tests.

Special proof tests

These are tests carried out specifically to prove the presence of NOHL, such tests not normally forming part of an audiological investigation. They may be merely extensions of conventional audiological tests or require quite different techniques and equipment. The former include use of ascending and descending threshold measurements in pure-tone threshold determination, the Stenger test, the Fournier technique in speech audiometry, and the use of reversed and converging sweeps in Békésy audiometry. All of these have been described above. The two special tests are delayed auditory feedback tests and electric response audiometry.

Delayed auditory feedback (DAF)

The principle of these tests is that the motor performance of a patient in such tasks as speaking or key-tapping can be disturbed if their acoustic signals (i.e. the patient's own voice or the tones resulting from the key-taps) are fed back to his ears with a time delay of between 100 ms and 250 ms. Unfortunately, many things go wrong with these tests, the most notable being that some patients are not affected by DAF at all, some are not affected except at levels that are perhaps 50 or 60 dB above threshold, and others habituate rapidly.

Delayed speech feedback (DSF) does not require elaborate or specialized equipment. A two-channel three-head tape recorder with a microphone for recording the patient's voice is sufficient, connected to an audiometer. The latter is used to monitor the speech input level, deliver the signal to either one or both earphones at the desired level, and put masking noise into the non-test earphone. The other requirement is that the signal being recorded can be fed into the audiometer directly, or played back into it as the tape passes from the recording head to the playback head. The distance between the two heads is commonly about 1.5 in (4 cm), and with a tape speed of 7.5 ips (about 20 cm/s), this gives a delay of about 200 ms between the spoken word and its playback.

The patient may be asked to read something out aloud, but apparently many NOHL patients cannot read properly! Some form of recitation has been found more suitable, and the difficulty of that task may have to be adjusted to the ability of the patient. We commonly ask the patient simply to repeat a series of 'one-two-three' sequences.

The effects of switching from synchronous to delayed feedback are various and include raising the voice (partly a Lombard effect), lowering the voice, speeding the voice, slowing the voice, slurring and stuttering. The results relate only to the threshold of hearing of speech and not to discrimination of speech; thus the test is not of much help in cases of high-tone hearing loss, such as that due to noise. Because of the wide range of normal values, quantitative interpretation of DSF test results is difficult. Occasionally, in a patient very sensitive to DSF, the test gives a fairly accurate indication of the true thresholds of hearing of speech, but in the majority of cases one cannot say more than that the patient's threshold for hearing of speech is not elevated beyond a certain level (the lowest level at which DSF effects were observed). Of course, where severe hearing loss is being feigned, the test may provide strong proof of the presence of NOHL. A demonstration of DSF may also help in management of the patient, as will be discussed in the final section of this chapter.

A pure-tone audiometer can be used to record the key tapping in what has been termed the 'delayed tone feedback tapping test' (DAFTT). In this the patient has to tap out a regular pattern of, for example, four beats alternating with two beats. First, the tapping rhythm is recorded on paper whilst there is simultaneous feedback of test tones. The feedback is then delayed and the new tapping rhythm recorded is compared with the synchronous record. Occasionally the response is quite dramatic and obvious. More often there are considerable irregularities in tapping rhythm for both delayed and synchronous feedback. Analysis would need on-line computer facilities if it is to be acceptably speedy and precise for clinical purposes. Moreover, in many instances there is rapid habituation to the disturbance of tapping rhythm. Our experience with this test soon led us to discard it, even before the advent of electric response audiometry, which, in any event, would have replaced the DAFTT test.

Electric response audiometry (ERA)

This can be defined as the measurement of electric responses from the auditory system to acoustic stimuli. It is objective in the sense that, like the acoustic reflex responses and DAF responses, these responses are not voluntary. On the other hand, there is usually a considerable element of operator-subjectivity in deciding whether a particular change in the ongoing EEG activity is acoustically evoked or not. Methods are being developed for removing or minimizing this element of subjectivity from ERA, but these are not yet widely available. The three main forms of ERA currently in clinical use are the 'slow' vertex responses, cochlear and eighth-nerve responses, and brain stem responses (listed in order of their development for such purposes).

TYPES OF ERA

The cortical or slow vertex responses are used principally for the objective measurement of pure-tone thresholds. They correspond closely to behavioural thresholds, but require a passively cooperative and awake patient. The responses arise from activation of wide areas of cerebral cortex and are a measure of the function of the whole auditory system, with the exception of the final stage of conscious perception and understanding the signal.

Electric responses at the other end of the auditory system are measured by electrocochleography (ECochG), commonly performed with a transtympanic electrode but sometimes with a non-invasive extratympanic electrode. Both techniques are used to measure the cochlear microphonics, summating potential and the eighth nerve action potential. These give quantitative information on the response of the cochlea and eighth cranial nerve, and also some differential diagnostic information. The stimulus is usually a broad-band click, but some limited frequency-specific information can be obtained with filtered clicks and other procedures. Recording can be carried out in anaesthetized, sedated or sleeping patients, and the procedure is thus suitable for children who are too hyperactive or sleepy for slow vertex response testing. Its value is, however, limited to measurement of peripheral auditory function and its frequency-specificity is limited. In its most common, transtympanic form, it is also invasive.

Although the risks of ECochG are small, they are not considered to be justifiable in medicolegal cases in which the reason for performing ERA is to obtain an objective measurement of threshold. The vertex responses are much more satisfactory in this respect. ECochG is used in some medicolegal cases, but in my view this should be reserved strictly for those cases where the physician has the patient's informed consent to assume a new role – that of medical practitioner responsible for the patient. In cases of alleged noise-induced hearing loss, for instance, ECochG is unlikely to provide worthwhile assistence to the physician in giving an expert opinion regarding the presence and extent of that condition that its use for legal purposes seems to be unjustified. There is also an ethical point to be considered here. The legal patient may feel that he has to comply with all the test requirements set out by the physician to whom he has been referred, or he may feel at some legal disadvantage if he does not comply. This militates further against the use of invasive, unpleasant or potentially harmful techniques, especially when they are not generally considered necessary for the diagnosis of the particular alleged injury.

The third main form of ERA is the measurement of the brain stem responses. Whilst these have a great potential diagnostic value, and can also be used for estimation of the true threshold, the actual voltages measured are rather small and the techniques are not yet fully frequency-specific. They are of great value in detecting neurological disorders, and particularly useful in children in whom invasive methods or techniques involving anaesthesia are undesirable and in those not suitable for vertex response tests. In legal cases, where it is desired to measure or estimate the threshold of hearing at several tone frequencies in each ear, and the patient is a passively cooperative adult, we agree with Alberti (1981b) that the vertex responses are the most satisfactory form of ERA.

INDICATIONS FOR ERA

Usually, ERA is carried out in legal contexts only when NOHL is suspected. Those who see medicolegal cases of deafness need to develop a high degree of awareness of NOHL in order to detect it readily, and regular use of ERA when they start such work will help this. It is also important to learn how to discourage the patient from exaggerating. A most effective means is to explain to him that noise-induced hearing loss has a particular pattern which will only become apparent if he responds faithfully to all the tones that he can hear, however weak they may be; and that, if he fails to do so, the hearing loss is liable to have the appearance of some other form of disorder which would not be attributable to noise damage.

Any large-scale scheme for settlement, e.g. a governmental scheme or one negotiated by a union for large numbers of its members scattered across the country, of necessity involves many otolaryngologists. With such schemes there is probably a case for having random ERA checks to act as a deterrent, and as a means of developing and maintaining ERA skills and building up an awareness of the prevalence and characteristics of NOHL. It may, however, be more cost-effective to use ERA in all cases where the apparent hearing loss in the compensation-assessment frequencies exceeds some substantial value, thereby preventing undeserved settlements for high figures.

In individual medicolegal cases, ERA may either be restricted to those in whom NOHL is suspected or it may be carried out routinely. The latter is advantageous generally and is my own practice. However, it does tend to be wasteful in cases with a hearing loss of typically noise-induced configuration and of such modest proportion that there can really be no question of NOHL. Enough has been said already on the various indicators of NOHL, but 'probably the most useful combination is a suspicious audiologist and a discrepancy between speech reception thresholds and pure-tone averages' (Alberti, Morgan and Le Blanc, 1974). To this, a further criterion can now be added (for alleged noise deafness cases), namely that ERA be used whenever the apparent sensorineural hearing loss at 500 Hz is greater than 35 dB (Alberti, Morgan and Czuba, 1978) or 25 dB (Coles, unpublished observation).

REQUIREMENTS OF MEDICOLEGAL ERA

Various types of hospital department give ERA services, but not all may be experienced in medicolegal work. The physician may therefore need to give precise guidance as to what he wants. The first point is to specify that it is the vertex responses which are required. The frequencies to be tested will need to be stated as far as possible, and I prefer to remain at least in telephone contact with the ERA department while tests are being done since the original requirements may have to be changed. Occasionally some further testing is indicated in order to clarify the position, e.g. to double-check discrepant results or add further test frequencies. This apart, ERA testing should be done 'blind', that is, the tester should not see the volunteered audiograms beforehand, or, if he does see them, not know whether they are likely to be correct or false. This tends to prevent bias in his identification of responses.

Because of time factors, tests are usually carried out in 10 dB steps with the minimum number of test frequencies. Commonly two frequencies in each ear are enough, although it may sometimes be preferable to test three frequencies in the better ear and only one in the other ear just to verify it. More frequencies may be needed for particular compensation formulae, or where NOHL is present and there is need to identify both the audiometric configuration and the degree of any underlying organic disorder.

There is a natural tendency for personnel carrying out ERA tests in medicolegal cases to apply too cautious criteria for fear of having to defend their opinion in cross-examination. This biases their estimates of threshold towards greater apparent hearing losses, which in turn has the unfortunate effect of biasing the award of damages in favour of the claimant. It is necessary, therefore, to give a 'best estimate' of the ERA thresholds, rather than a statement of the lowest level at which responses were quite definitely obtained. Moreover, the tester should interpret between the 10 dB steps to the nearest 5 dB in order to allow proper comparison with the volunteered thresholds and with the form of audiometric measurements from which most compensation scales have been derived.

INTERPRETATION OF RESULTS

ERA results usually fall quite easily into one of two categories. Either they correspond reasonably closely to the volunteered thresholds or they show hearing thresholds markedly more acute than those volunteered. Up to now, I have used the following criteria to judge whether or not ERA responses corroborate the volunteered ones. Where several frequencies have been measured in one ear, the objective/subjective differences are averaged and if they exceed about 10 dB the results are regarded as discrepant. For one individual test frequency, an ERA threshold of up to 20 dB more acute is regarded as suspicious, but not necessarily proof of NOHL.

If the ERA results are taken as corroborating the volunteered ones, then the volunteered ones are used for compensation assessment. That is, if the person's volunteered responses are truthful, they (and not the ERA) express what he actually hears, which in turn defines his auditory ability or disability. However, when the volunteered responses are shown to be false, the ERA values are used for calculating the disability.

ANALYSIS OF RESULTS

The results of 467 routine ERA tests (209 ears) in a consecutive series of 118 medicolegal cases seen in Nottingham from October 1979 to December 1981 have been analysed. These were all taking private legal action against their employers for damages arising out of alleged noise-induced hearing loss and/or tinnitus. The distribution of differences between objective (ERA) and corresponding subjective (conventional manual audiometry) measurements is shown in *Figure 10.4*. There

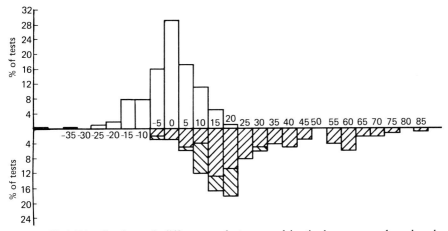

Figure 10.4 Distribution of differences between objectively measured and volunteered thresholds: organic and non-organic medicolegal cases. (Total N = 118 patients, 6 of whom had organic HL in one ear and NOHL in the other). (Positive values refer to lower thresholds when tested objectively). □ = organic cases (*n* = 362 tests in 167 ears of 99 patients); ▨ = NOHL detected before ERA (*n* = 82 tests in 27 ears of 19 patients); ▧ = NOHL not detected before ERA (*n* = 23 tests in 11 ears of 6 patients)

were three categories of patients: (a) those without signs of NOHL at any stage, (b) NOHL revealed by ERA only, and (c) NOHL indicated before ERA and confirmed by it. In no cases was NOHL thought to be present and then disproved by ERA. But in 178 ears considered to have wholly organic hearing loss, non-organic loss was later found by ERA in 11 (6%), which confirms the desirability of routine use of ERA in medicolegal work.

The extent of the exaggeration in the NOHL cases can be seen, but there is some overlap in the two distributions in the −5 dB to a +20 dB range. This of course refers to single-frequency tests; in most cases these were followed by tests at other frequencies when the average showed either more consistent discrepancy from or agreement with the volunteered thresholds.

For individual tests, the limits of the agreement between objective and subjective data in organic cases are usually ± 15 dB, with an occasional value of +20 dB or −20 dB or more. The data have also been analysed for all those cases where three or more tests were carried out in one ear. In 89 cases showing organic hearing loss, three to five tests (mean 3.9) were carried out and the averaged objective/ subjective difference exceeded 7.5 dB in only 3 cases. In 19 cases showing NOHL, three to seven tests (mean 5.7) were carried out and the averaged difference failed to exceed 7.5 dB in only one. Clearly, a 7.5 dB criterion would be most useful for clinical and medicolegal purposes. Similar degrees of precision have been reported by Alberti (1970) in a control group tested in the environment of 'a busy routine clinical unit'.

The question remains whether there is some general shift in medicolegal cases towards exaggeration of the hearing loss, additional to those cases found to have an identifiable NOHL overlay. Happily, the Nottingham Department of Medical Physics have carried out a study of objective/subjective differences in audiometric threshold of persons with normal hearing or organic hearing disorders (Mason, Su and Hayes, 1977). Their ERA equipment and techniques were comparable to those used in the present series, although somewhat less sophisticated. The mean value of the difference was −1.7 dB, the objectively determined thresholds being slightly less acute than the volunteered (subjective) ones. This figure agrees well with that found in the present series (−0.8 dB), and with the −2.2 dB measured by Davis (1964) and the data published by Beagley (1973), the last two series showing a distribution of differences skewed in the direction of a few objective thresholds which are markedly less acute than the corresponding subjective ones. A few such values (three of −25 dB, one of −35 dB, and one of −60 dB) were also found in patients without NOHL in the present series, and several further such discrepancies have been seen since. Some of them were due to high levels of background electrical activity in the brain, but in others there was no evident explanation. The discrepancies were not related to test frequency.

The distribution of the data of Mason, Su and Hayes (1977) and of Davis (1964) is shown in *Figure 10.5*, each compared to that of the organic cases in the present medicolegal series. There is no significant difference between the three series, but visual examination of the distribution might suggest 5 or 10 dB of exaggeration in about 5% of the tests. If that is true, then it may have to be accepted that there is occasional slight exaggeration that ERA does not detect.

COMPARISON OF ADULT AND CHILD CASES OF NOHL

Children and adults with NOHL tend to show somewhat different patterns of response in audiometric tests. Three explanations seem possible. The child may be less able to exaggerate convincingly, he may be less skilful at audiometry in general, or he may be more influenced by the degree to which the audiometric task

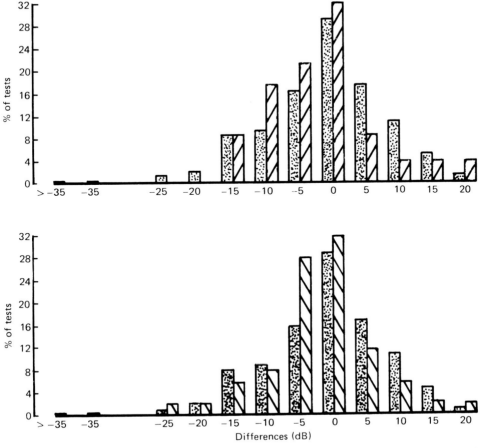

Figure 10.5 Distribution of differences between objectively measured and volunteered thresholds: organic medicolegal cases compared with controls (Mason, Su and Hayes, 1977) and another group (Davis, 1964). (Positive values refer to lower thresholds when tested objectively). ⊡ = Coles, organic cases (*n* = 362 tests); ▨ = Mason, Su and Hayes. (*n* = 24 tests); ▧ = Davis (*n* = 50 tests)

interests him. To study this difference in performance, a special analysis has been made of patients with symmetrical hearing loss (both apparent and true), who obviously have no auditory reference point, i.e. no normal or relatively normal ear. Sixty cases met these selection criteria, 32 of them adults and 28 children.

In the pure-tone a-c tests, there was little difference in performance between children and adults, the children being perhaps slightly less reliable (*Table 10.2*). However, *Table 10.3* shows that more acute thresholds were indicated by b-c than a-c in a very much higher proportion of children than adults, even after exclusion of cases in whom otoscopy and/or acoustic impedance and reflex tests had shown a middle ear disorder. Speech audiometry showed even greater differences between children and adults, particularly where results were at, or closer to, the true threshold (*Table 10.4*).

If the first hypothesis, i.e. that children are less skilled when it comes to exaggeration, was correct, one might expect greater differences between adults and children in pure-tone a-c test performance. One would also expect similar differences in the other tests. Instead, the data are interpreted as supporting the third hypothesis, i.e. that NOHL in children is more commonly due to inattention.

Table 10.2 Comparison of adults and children with symmetrical NOHL: performance in pure-tone air-conduction audiometry (PTA) (1972–77 sample)

	Adults	*Children*
PTA variable and/or imprecise	21 (66%)	22 (79%)
PTA repeatable and precise	11 (34%)	6 (21%)
Total	32	28

Table 10.3 Comparison of adults and children with symmetrical NOHL: prevalence of apparent air/bone gaps* (1972–77 sample)

	Adults	*Children*
Apparent a/b gap (but no middle ear disorder present)	2 (6%)	12 (43%)
a/b gap indicated (and a middle ear disorder present)	4 (13%)	5 (18%)
No a/b gap indicated	26 (81%)	11 (39%)
Total	32	28

* An air/bone (a/b) gap is defined here as being present when the average b-c thresholds are better than the average of the corresponding a-c ones by at least 20 dB.

Table 10.4 Comparison of adults and children with symmetrical NOHL: performance in speech audiometry (1972–77 sample)

	Adults	*Children*
Speech thresholds true	17 (53%)	24 (86%)
Speech thresholds better (but not true)	10 (31%)	4 (14%)
Speech thresholds consistent with pure-tone ones	5 (16%)	0
Speech thresholds worse	0	0
Total	32	28

MANAGEMENT OF THE PATIENT SHOWING NOHL

The majority of cases need little in the way of treatment, further investigation or other management. Nevertheless, something has to be said to the patient.

In medicolegal cases it is better to let a man 'off the hook' rather than make him lose face and perhaps become obstinate or even aggressive. He is much more likely to accept the reduced financial settlement which is his due if the audiometric discrepancies are explained to him as a probable misunderstanding of the response task required of him in ordinary audiometry. If he has given a history of marked auditory disability, then this can be attributed (often quite truthfully) to a loss of confidence in his ability to hear soft sounds or hear clearly. Often the excess disability disappears once the legal case has been settled one way or another.

In the occasional case of apparently severe auditory disability, albeit without organic cause, it is often helpful to tell the patient and/or his family that he really *can* hear quite well but has lost confidence in this, and then to demonstrate this by means of delayed speech feedback. The effect is first demonstrated to the relatives who try out DSF for themselves, and explained to all those present, including the patient. The patient is then tested, and the evident effect of DSF is pointed out to him and his relatives. It should be explained to him that he must have heard the delayed feedback for it to have had the observed effect on his voice production. Very rarely has the author felt it necessary to refer the patient to a psychiatrist.

If the patient has been given a hearing aid and is making considerable use of it, it is sometimes better to leave him with it as a 'prop' until he builds up confidence. Sooner or later he will forget to put it on, find he can hear without it, and gradually cease to use it.

The child has to be let 'off the hook' somewhat differently. Obviously the parents have to be informed of the true state of his hearing. It is also necessary to explain that it is not the child's 'fault', or that the exaggeration is very understandable and not at all uncommon in view of the circumstances (whatever these may be). The parents should be warned not to castigate, tease or punish the child, but simply treat him as normal (or according to his true hearing ability) and forget the whole incident as soon as possible. The child should be told what his hearing state is and that his parents are aware of this. He, too, soon forgets his simulated deafness if he is allowed to.

SUMMARY

Non-organic hearing loss remains with us as an ever-present differential diagnosis or overlay in clinical otological/audiological practice. In more recent years it has assumed greater importance in many countries because of increasing awareness of noise as an industrial hazard, which in turn has resulted in an increase in claims for compensation for noise-induced hearing loss. The present chapter reviews the subject of NOHL in both general clinical and medicolegal contexts. The most important ingredients for detection of NOHL and measurement of the true hearing thresholds are; (1) otological and audiological staff alert to the problem and observant of the many ways in which the NOHL case may reveal his true identity; (2) critical use of well-calibrated speech audiometry, and of acoustic impedance and reflex tests; and (3) ready availability of electric response audiometry measuring the slow vertex potentials, particularly for medicolegal cases.

Acknowledgements

I wish to thank the many colleagues who have assisted me at Southampton and Nottingham in the clinical work which has formed the basis of the material presented here. In particular, I acknowledge the help of Dr V. M. Priede (Institute of Sound and Vibration Research, University of Southampton) and Mr S. M. Mason and Dr K. Bradshaw (Department of Medical Physics, University Hospital, Nottingham.)

References

Alberti, P. W. (1970) New tools for old tricks. *Annals of Otology, Rhinology and Laryngology*, **79**, 800–807

Alberti, P. W. (1981a) Compensation for industrial hearing loss: the practice in Canada. In *Audiology and Audiological Medicine*, edited by H. A. Beagley, pp. 880–895. London and Oxford: Oxford University Press

Alberti, P. W. (1981b) Non-organic hearing loss in adults. In *Audiology and Audiological Medicine*, edited by H. A. Beagley, pp. 910–931. London and Oxford: Oxford University Press

Alberti, P. W., Morgan, P. P. and Czuba, I. (1978) Speech and puretone audiometry as a screen for exaggerated hearing loss in industrial claims. *Acta Oto-Laryngologica*, **87**, 728–731

Alberti, P. W., Morgan, P. P. and Le Blanc, J. C. (1974) Occupational hearing loss: an otologist's view of a long-term study. *Laryngoscope*, **84**, 1822–1834

Anderson, H. and Wedenberg, E. (1968) Audiometric identification of normal hearing carriers of genes for deafness. *Acta Oto-Laryngologica*, **65**, 535–554

Beagley, H. A. (1973) Electrophysiological methods in the diagnosis and management of deafness. *Minerva Otorhinolaringologica*, **23**, 173–181

Borg, E. (1973) On the neuronal organisation of the acoustic middle-ear reflex. A physiological and anatomical study. *Brain Research*, **49**, 101–123

Coles, R. R. A. (1967) External meatus closure by audiometer earphone. *Journal of Speech and Hearing Disorders*, **32**, 296–297

Coles, R. R. A., Markides, A. and Priede, V. M. (1973) Uses and abuses of speech audiometry. In *Disorders of Auditory Function*, edited by W. Taylor, pp. 181–202. London: Academic Press

Coles, R. R. A. and Priede, V. M. (1970) On the misdiagnoses arising from incorrect use of masking. *Journal of Laryngology and Otology*, **84**, 41–63

Coles, R. R. A. and Priede, V. M. (1971) Non-organic overlay in noise-induced hearing loss. *Proceedings of the Royal Society of Medicine*, **64**, 194–199

Coles, R. R. A. and Priede, V. M. (1976) Speech discrimination tests in investigation of sensorineural hearing loss. *Journal of Laryngology and Otology*, **90**, 1081–1092

Corcoran, A. L., Cleaver, V. C. G. and Stephens, S. D. G. (1980) Attention, eye closure and the acoustic reflex. *Audiology*, **19**, 233–244

Davis, H. (1964) Slow cortical evoked potentials. *Acta Oto-Laryngologica*, Suppl. 206, 128–134

Doerfler, L. G. (1951) Psychogenic deafness and its detection. *Annals of Otology, Rhinology and Laryngology*, **68**, 1045–1048

Fournier, J. E. (1956) La dépistage de la simulation auditive. In *Exposés Annuels d'Oto-Rhino-Laryngologie*, pp. 107–126. Paris: Masson et Cie. (Also translation No. 8 (1958) of the Beltone Institute for Hearing Research, Chicago: The detection of auditory malingering)

Goldstein, R. (1967) Pseudohypacusis. *Journal of Speech and Hearing Disorders*, **31**, 341–352

Green, D. S. (1978) Pure tone air-conduction testing. In *Handbook of Clinical Audiology*, edited by J. Katz, pp. 98–109. Baltimore: Williams & Wilkins

Harris, D. A. (1958) A rapid and simple technique for the detection of non-organic hearing loss. *Archives of Otolaryngology*, **68**, 758–760

Hyde, M. L., Alberti, P. W., Morgan, P. P., Symons, F. and Cummings, F. (1980) Puretone threshold estimations from acoustic reflex thresholds: a myth? *Acta Oto-Laryngologica*, **89**, 345–357

Jerger, J. (1960) Békésy audiometry in analysis of auditory disorders. *Journal of Speech and Hearing Research*, **3**, 275–287

Jerger, J., Burney, P., Mauldin, L. and Crump, B. (1974) Predicting hearing loss from the acoustic reflex. *Journal of Speech and Hearing Disorders*, **39**, 11–22

Jerger, J., Hayes, D. and Anthony, L. (1978) Effect of age on prediction of sensorineural hearing level from the acoustic reflex. *Archives of Otolaryngology*, **104**, 393–394

Jerger, J. and Herer, G. (1961) Unexpected dividend in Békésy audiometry. *Journal of Speech and Hearing Disorders*, **26**, 390–391

Johnsen, J. D., Osterhammel, D., Terkildsen, K., Osterhammel, P. and Huis in't Velt, F. (1976) The white noise middle ear muscle reflex threshold in patients with sensorineural hearing impairment. *Scandinavian Audiology*, **5**, 131–135

Kerr, A. G., Gillespie, W. J. and Easton, J. M. (1975) Deafness: a simple test for malingering. *British Journal of Audiology*, **9**, 24–26

Markides, A. (1980) The relation between hearing loss for pure tones and hearing loss for speech among hearing-impaired children. *British Journal of Audiology*, **14**, 115–121

Mason, S. M., Su, A. P. and Hayes, R. A. (1977) Simple online detector of auditory evoked cortical potentials. *Medical and Biological Engineering and Computing*, **15**, 641–647

Metz, O. (1952) Threshold of reflex contractions of muscles of middle ear and recruitment of loudness. *Archives of Otolaryngology*, **55**, 536–543

Niemeyer, W. and Sesterhenn, G. (1974) Calculating the hearing threshold from the stapedius reflex threshold for different sound stimuli. *Audiology*, **13**, 421–427

Priede, V. M. (1973) Study of tests for differentiating between sensory and peripheral neural types of auditory dysfunctions. *PhD Thesis*, University of Southampton

Priede, V. M. and Coles, R. R. A. (1974) Interpretation of loudness recruitment tests: some new concepts and criteria. *Journal of Laryngology and Otology*, **88,** 641–662

Sesterhenn, G. and Breuninger, H. (1977) Determination of hearing threshold for single frequencies from the acoustic reflex. *Audiology*, **16,** 201–214

Shammas, E. N. (1974) Studies on the technique and interpretation of the pure-tone Stenger test. *MSc Dissertation*, University of Southampton

Smith, B. L. and Markides, A. (1981) Interaural attenuation for pure tones and speech. *British Journal of Audiology*, **15,** 49–54

Snyder, J. M. (1973) Interaural attenuation characteristics in audiometry. *Laryngoscope*, **83,** 1847–1855

Terkildsen, K., Osterhammel, P. and Bretlau, P. (1973) Acoustic middle-ear muscle reflexes in patients with otosclerosis. *Archives of Otolaryngology*, **98,** 152–155

11
Physiological basis of diagnosis and treatment of the dizzy patient
Brian F. McCabe

THE IMPORTANCE OF THE HISTORY

In the diagnosis of the dizzy patient, the first problem, or fork in the flow sheet, is distinguishing between vestibular and extravestibular sources of the symptom. Extravestibular dizziness is far more common than the vestibular kind, and the single best tool to distinguish between the two is the history. A physician who develops the art of history-taking to a high degree has a great advantage over one who depends primarily upon physical findings and laboratory tests. Otolaryngologists tend to rely on their highly developed ability to peer into the nooks and crannies of the head and neck, and may develop an attitude that 'if you can't see it, the patient hasn't got it'. Nowhere is such an attitude less helpful than in diagnosing the dizzy patient for whom the physical examination and laboratory tests, including audiometry and electronystagmography (ENG) are frequently normal. When the physician hears the complaint 'Doctor, I'm dizzy', he knows he is committed to a protracted investigation before he can make even a differential diagnosis. The initial and single most important part of this investigation is the history.

The history must be total, encompassing present illness, past medical history, surgical history, family history, drug history, allergic history, social and work history, trauma history, and system review. An adequate history on initial work-up takes, on the average, one hour or longer. In a clinical practice it may be necessary to take the history *en bloc*, with indicated tests interspersed. It is far better to do it this way, if necessary, than to truncate the time to fit one's schedule of patients. Too often, once the initial history is taken, further historical questions are never asked, with the result that promising leads are never followed. The patient has so little insight into the disease and the symptoms are so complex (vestibular complaints are almost always multisystem in origin) that he may not volunteer important information, which must be specifically extracted from him.

To give an exhaustive example of a composite history is impossible in these few pages; it would require a volume. We can, however, cite a few examples of a helpful and productive beginning of the history. Basic to the history are two attributes with which the physician must be equipped:

(1) He must have knowledge of how the vestibular system (central and peripheral) operates. For example, if unconsciousness is part of the dizzy spell, the disease cannot be vestibular. The vestibular system does not work that way. At this point, then, the first big fork in the flow sheet, the problem of distinguishing vestibular from non-vestibular origins, may be passed.

(2) He must be cognizant of the clinical features of all the diseases that cause dizziness. For example, if the physician has not heard of vestibular migraine and does not know at least its clinical characteristics, he will never diagnose it. Many patients have great difficulty typifying their dizziness, even the chief complaint. They must frequently be led, but in a non-directive way. An important initial distinction is between vertigo (patients do not say, 'Doctor, I've got vertigo') and non-vertiginous dizziness. An excellent example of non-directive leading is for the physician to ask the patient to describe the dizziness without using the word 'dizzy'. The patient may then describe the room moving round and round or the pictures on the wall moving right to left, and true vertigo is established. Or the patient describes the dizziness as floating on air, and the possibility of psychic dizziness enters the differential diagnosis. (We are indebted to Dr Hugh Barber for this bit of advice.)

Another example of historical refinement is the distinction between ataxia and spontaneous spells. Patients will seldom volunteer that their dizziness is present only on locomotion and never on sitting, standing, or lying still. When spontaneous, precipitators of spells must be sought: a certain position or change in position; a particular position of the head or the neck, e.g. consistently looking over one shoulder on backing up the car (cervical vertigo?); time of day (hypoglycemia?); relationship to the menstrual cycle; drug use (the *Physicians Desk Reference* can be helpful); and presence or absence of an aura or other neurological events, such as sensory or motor problems, before, during, or after the spell. These are some of the more important features of the history which need to be elicited from the patient.

The physician may frequently be misled or confused in diagnosis by failing to identify the patient as having two kinds of spells. This may lead to (1) misdiagnosis, (2) diagnosis of two conditions when only one is present, or (3) failure to diagnose two coexisting diseases. An example of the second is the combination of typical Ménière's attacks and spontaneous momentary spells of collapse, referred to as 'falling spells of Tumarkin'. These spells may be confused with transient ischemic attacks (TIAs) and lead one away from the proper diagnosis to one of brain stem ischemia. They are definitely vestibular in origin, and are a dramatic example of the powerful effect the vestibulospinal tracts can have on the motor system. An example of failure to diagnose two coexisting diseases is the not infrequent coexistence of peripheral polyneuronitis of the lower extremities and central (e.g. toxic alcoholic cerebellitis) or end-organ disease.

VESTIBULAR PHYSIOLOGY FOR THE CLINICIAN

The anatomy and physiology of the vestibular system are important to the student, interesting to the clinician, and essential to the researcher. It is important to the

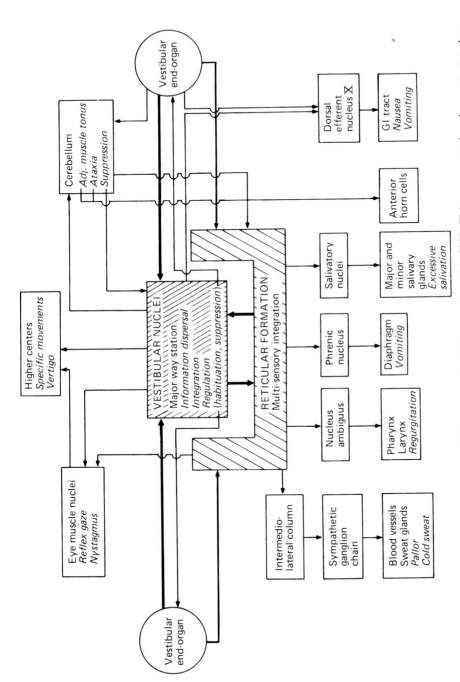

Figure 11.1 The vestibular system is two-sided, constantly discharging into the CNS. This representation demonstrates the processing of normal and abnormal impulses, and the extremely high degree to which the vestibular system is integrated into the neuraxis. (From McCabe, Ryu and Sekitani, 1972, courtesy of the Editors and Publishers, *Laryngoscope*, **82**, 231. Further experiments on vestibular compensation)

student to know how the basic components of this system work, and how the system interacts with others as a basis for understanding the pathophysiology of vestibular disease. It is interesting to the clinician to see what a marvelously constructed and integrated system this is. It would be overstating the case, however, to claim that extensive anatomical and physiological knowledge is essential, or even helpful, to understanding the manifestations or aberrations of the system. Rather than knowing and remembering brain tracts, Ewald's second law, and the types of endings on the hair cell, a conceptual knowledge of the system's organization and how it works is clinically helpful. An overview of the vestibular system's integration into the neuraxis (presented as a block diagram in *Figure 11.1*), including the terms of functional interrelation, is more meaningful than the presentation and study of brain tracts.

A simplified concept of function

The endolymphatic system consists of the coiling cochlear duct at one end, three semicircular ducts at the other, and three specializations of this continuous tube in between: the utricle, the saccule, and the endolymphatic duct and sac. Any movement of the head in which there is some angular acceleration causes an accumulation of endolymph on one side of the cupulae of two or more of the six semicircular canals (they are orthogonally paired structures), and the brain is signaled. The density of the cupula and endolymph is probably the same, since their refractive indices are the same. Hence, gravity cannot affect the cupulae. The utricle and the saccule contain flat sensory areas, and the maculae, overlaid by a gelatinous coat studded with calcified bodies, contain the otoliths. These organs appear best equipped to sense linear acceleration, of which gravity is one variety.

The vestibular end-organs are dynamic structures. They are dynamic in three ways:

(1) They respond to linear and angular accelerations.
(2) They are not silent until stimulated but constantly discharge a resting pattern of signals to the brain (*Figure 11.2*). Acceleration or a change in acceleration deviates the cupula and produces a change in this pattern of signals (*Figure 11.3*); it is this change that is distributed to the brain and interpreted.
(3) There are two sets of vestibular systems, each constantly signaling. A difference in the signal pattern between right and left is produced by an acceleration, and it is this difference that is the relevant quantity to the brain (*Figure 11.4*).

The balance theory

The vestibular system, being an extremely old system phylogenetically, has diffuse connections with the CNS (*see Figure 11.1*). Some of the important areas upon which the vestibular system discharges are illustrated in *Figure 11.5* on a conceptual, rather than anatomical, basis. On normal stimulation there is a precise and

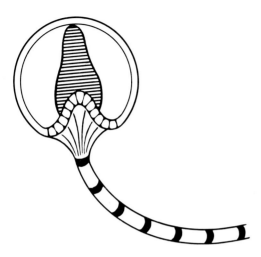

Figure 11.2 Ampullated end of one semicircular canal, showing the crista capped by the cupula and the vestibular nerve branch supplying it. Black bars represent impulse bursts along the nerve. Each end-organ has a resting discharge so that it is not silent at rest but has an 'open line' to the CNS. (From McCabe, 1973, Vestibular physiology: its clinical application in understanding the dizzy patient. In *Otolaryngology*, **1,** edited by M. M. Paparella and V. A. Shumrick, p. 318. Philadelphia: W. B. Saunders, courtesy of the Publishers)

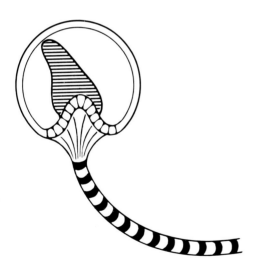

Figure 11.3 The crista is the frequency modulator of the resting discharge of its vestibular nerve. The cupula is deviated to the left, and the resting frequency is modulated upward to the exact degree of deviation. When the cupula is deviated to the right in this canal, the resting frequency will be modulated downward, proportionate to the degree of deviation. (From McCabe, 1973, Vestibular physiology: its clinical application in understanding the dizzy patient. In *Otolaryngology*, **1,** edited by M. M. Paparella and V. A. Shumrick, p. 318. Philadelphia: W. B. Saunders, courtesy of the Publishers)

182

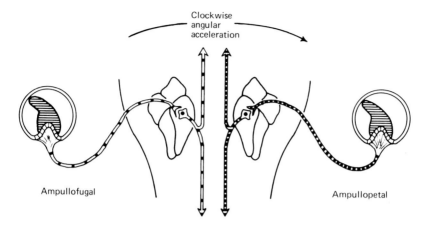

Figure 11.4 Two-sided vestibular system, which constantly discharges a proportionately equal and opposite message to the CNS. Modulation of the discharge above the resting level on the left is of a specific quantity; its paired canal on the right experiences an opposite endolymph flow of the same magnitude, resulting in modulation of the discharge below the resting level. This equal-and-opposite pattern is distributed to the brain and interpreted

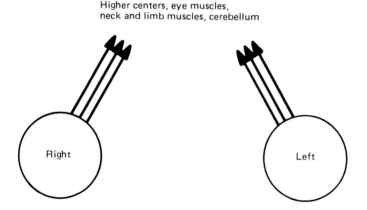

Figure 11.5 Balance theory of vestibular function: equilibrium. The two end-organs constantly discharge at steady state when at rest. On actuation, the brain receives impulses from both sides simultaneously, weighs one against the other, interprets the equal and opposite difference in discharge strength according to past experience, and transmits information. Each effector organ responds to its particular ability (e.g. awareness of motion, deviation of eyes to retain field of last gaze). (From McCabe, 1973, Vestibular physiology; its clinical application in understanding the dizzy patient. In *Otolaryngology*, **1,** edited by M. M. Paparella and V. A. Shumrick, p. 318. Philadelphia: W. B. Saunders, courtesy of the Publishers)

specific change in impulse patterns on the two sides. On one side the resting potential is modulated downward, and on the other side the resting discharge is modulated upward. As far as we know, the difference between the downward modulation on one side and the upward modulation on the other side is precisely the same. Thus, the two sides of the brain are informed in an equal but opposite manner. This polarity is important in understanding the system; the equality is even more important.

The numerous areas to which the vestibular system discharges respond in recognition (*see Figure 11.1*). The cerebral cortex interprets the change as movement of specific direction and speed. To compensate, the eye muscle nuclei move the eyes to retain the field of last gaze, opposite to the motion of the head; this acts as a protective mechanism in retaining orientation to environment. The anterior horn cells in the spinal cord adjust trunk and limb muscles, and the cerebellum adjusts muscle tonus to meet the new situation. These processes are probably partly instinctual and partly learned. The cortex, for example, most likely underwent a prolonged period of training while the organism was learning to stand and walk. It learned to match a certain degree of cupula displacement in response to sudden head motion to a specific degree of alteration of the surrounding environment by matching a number of modalities against it; for example, the eyes informed the brain that the body had moved so far, the proprioceptors informed the brain that the body had moved so far, and tactile modalities informed the brain when the organism had hit the floor. Over the years, the brain had learned exactly what to expect from its vestibular end-organs in combination with other modalities. Being a superb computer, the brain had integrated these sensations to a high degree by early childhood.

It is important to conceive the vestibular apparatus as two systems, right and left, in constant dynamic balance, one checking against the other, working as a team to inform the organism of movements and head positions, and adjusting the body to meet these new conditions.

It is also important to understand each vestibular system, right and left, as a complete, two-sided, and integrated system extending from end-organ to cortex, and not as an isolated end-organ on one side.

DISEASE STRIKES

When a sudden pathological diminution of function of one vestibular system occurs (vestibular crises are usually of the diminution or destructive rather than the irritative variety), e.g. a Ménière's spell of one end-organ, a major imbalance exists (*Figure 11.6*). The involved side is no longer able to deliver its equal and opposite fund of information to the brain. The two systems are discharging at rest at an unequal intensity, and unequal intensity of discharges has a specific meaning to the brain. The sequelae of this imbalance are manifestations of a relative hyperfunction of the intact side; thus, uncontrolled and prolonged vestibular reflexes result.

The disparate message arrives at the cerebral cortex, which interprets this unbalanced information from the two sides in the only way it can, i.e. based on past

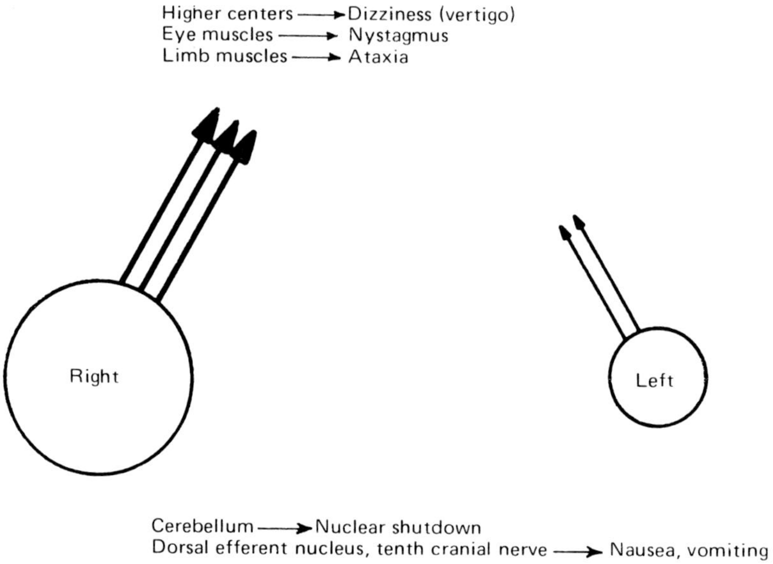

Higher centers ⟶ Dizziness (vertigo)
Eye muscles ⟶ Nystagmus
Limb muscles ⟶ Ataxia

Right

Left

Cerebellum ⟶ Nuclear shutdown
Dorsal efferent nucleus, tenth cranial nerve ⟶ Nausea, vomiting

Figure 11.6 Diminution of discharge caused by disease in the left labyrinth: crisis. (From McCabe, 1973, Vestibular physiology: its clinical application in understanding the dizzy patient. In *Otolaryngology*, **1**, edited by M. M. Paparella and V. A. Shumrick, p. 318. Philadelphia: W. B. Saunders, courtesy of the Publishers)

experience. The cortex interprets it as a condition of constant motion, and this is our definition of vertigo. This misinterpretation of the actual condition is a rotary sensation when the whole end-organ is involved, because the six semicircular canals predominate in their overall effects over misinformation from the four otolith organs alone, simply by the law of mass action. Thus, the sensation may be of a pitching, yawing, or rolling character but is always of a rotational nature because of this predominance of innervation.

The same massive imbalance in discharges arrives at the eye muscle nuclei and the reticular formation. The imbalance, interpreted, as before, in the light of past information and training, directs the eye muscle nuclei to deviate the eyes in the direction of last gaze to retain orientation; the slow component of nystagmus is born. The eyes, however, cannot continue to track indefinitely in any single direction because of their anatomical limitations. After a deviation specific to the number of motoneurons has occurred, inhibitor neurons in the reticular formation cut off the incoming flow from the vestibular nuclei and, at the same time, reticular activating neurons direct the ocular muscle nuclei to return the eyeball to the point of gaze at which the slow component began the deviation (across the midline). This second phase of eye deviation is much faster, because it is a compensatory or recovery phase. The quick component of nystagmus is thus generated. The reticular activating neuron, having fired, enters into its refractory period, and the end-organ inflow from the vestibular nuclei resumes its effect upon the eye muscle tracts: the eyeballs are directed again to retain the field of last gaze. This repetitive attempt to retain last field of gaze by a conjugate movement of the eyes and a rapid reflex return of the eyeballs across the midline in compensation is our definition of vestibular nystagmus.

The same imbalance of information is transmitted from the vestibular nuclei down the spinal cord to anterior horn cells, instructing the postural and locomotor muscles to meet a new situation that never occurs; staggering and ataxia result.

The imbalance in impulses also plays upon the dorsal efferent nucleus of the tenth cranial nerve. At first, this nucleus effects only a cessation of peristalsis. Gut activity is not needed in an emergent situation. If the imbalance is massive and continuous, however, this nucleus is heavily stimulated, and reverse peristalsis occurs, with resultant nausea and vomiting.

The effects mediated by the cerebellum in response to a massive imbalance on the two sides are only beginning to be understood. In a matter of minutes, the cerebellum imposes a virtual shutdown of electrical activity of the vestibular nuclei (at least the medial nucleus, the major way station for incoming canal impulses) by virtue of its profound inhibitory influence on vestibular activity (*Figure 11.7*). The cerebellum does not eliminate the great imbalance by this shutdown, because not all information from the end-organ distributes to the brain through these nuclei. Some fibers from the end-organ distribute straight to numerous other parts of the brain stem and cerebellum (*see Figure 11.1*) without vestibular nuclear synapse. The nuclear shutdown does not then eliminate the problem, but it does lessen the imbalance so that the full effects do not distribute through all available vestibular pathways.

The organism then sets about trying to restore the situation which it cannot long endure. It will eventually die through dehydration and fluid and electrolyte imbalance. Restoration of equilibrium between the two centers brings about resolution of the uncontrolled reflexes. This can be done in three ways: (1) restoration to health of the diseased system, which may take hours to days; (2) central suppression of the intact side by invocation of inhibitory tracts in the CNS; and (3) generation of a new electrical activity in the underdischarging system in order to balance the normal, but now relatively hyperactive, side (*Figure 11.8*). These include probably all theoretical mechanisms involved.

In practice, it is likely that all three mechanisms occur at once in varying degrees. For example, in the crisis of Ménière's disease the end-organ heals itself in a few hours, and a normal or near-normal discharge pattern from the end-organ resumes. The cerebellar clamp is not needed, or at least only temporarily. Reflexes then revert to normal, as equal and opposite reactions are signaled from the two end-organs.

Another example is acute suppurative labyrinthitis. In this disease the end-organ is destroyed, and, since it cannot rebuild itself, restoration must be a central process. Quickly the cerebellum imposes vestibular and nuclear shutdown, and this provides a barely tolerable situation for the organism as long as there is no, or at least only minimal, stimulation of the opposite end-organ to accentuate the great imbalance. For this reason, patients in vestibular crisis remain perfectly still, with as little head motion as possible. Movement of the head results in accentuation of the imbalance, with waves of vertigo and vegetative symptoms. Then, over a matter of days and possibly weeks, a new resting electrical activity is generated in the

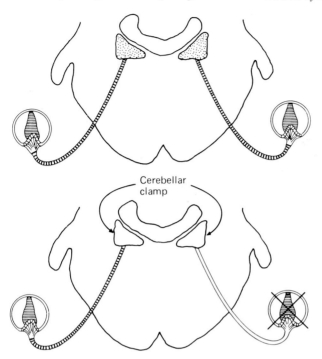

Figure 11.7 Results of massive imbalance. At rest, discharges from each end-organ result in a certain level of activity in the medial vestibular nucleus of each side, represented by the quantity of dots in each nucleus (*top*). With a severe lesion of one end-organ, sufficient to deprive its nerve of resting discharges and the ability to respond, the cerebellum, which has direct connections not only with nuclei but with each end-organ, applies a clamp which during the critical period of recovery or compensation renders each nucleus electrically silent (*bottom*). This does not eliminate symptoms (vestibular interconnections are too wide-spread), but does redress the situation by rebalancing part of the vestibular system at a lower level of activity. This lessens the impact of massive imbalance on the rest of the neuraxis. The clamp will be slowly released as new resting activity is generated in the deprived nucleus. (From McCabe, 1973, Vestibular physiology: its clinical application in understanding the dizzy patient. In *Otolaryngology*, **1,** edited by M. M. Paparella and V. A. Shumrick, p. 318. Philadelphia: W. B. Saunders, courtesy of the Publishers)

denervated vestibular nuclei. As this new activity builds up, symptoms abate and the cerebellar shutdown is slowly released. When this activity is fully restored and matches the other side, symptoms disappear, except for varying degrees of motion intolerance. Motion interpretation involves integration, and this must gradually be built up following regeneration of resting activity in the nuclei.

We do not know what stimulates the generation of the new resting activity in the denervated nuclei, but we know of certain requisites for it. Certainly there must be a chronic vestibular input imbalance or, more simply, a vacuum stimulating its need. The speed at which generation is brought about is dependent upon the severity of the imbalance stimulating it and the ability of the CNS to respond. This ability is a function of the vigor of the whole organism, affected by the age of the patient, availability of neuron arcs, and efficiency of the CNS vascular supply.

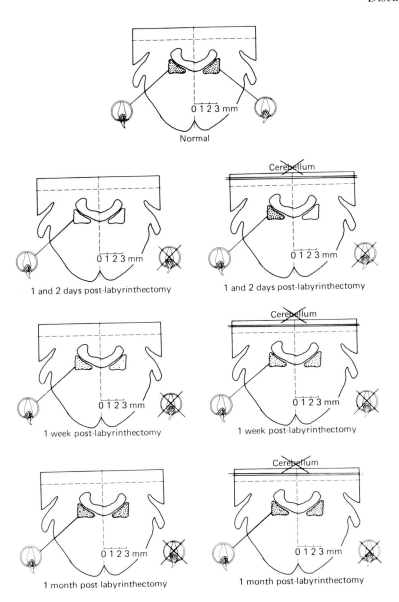

Figure 11.8 Brain stem sections at the level of the medial vestibular nuclei. The number of dots within each medial nucleus outline indicates the proportionate amount of electrical activity in the animal. At 1 and 2 days after labyrinthectomy there was profound damping of electrical activity of both nuclei. Cerebellectomy produces awakening to normal or near-normal levels of electrical activity on the contralateral side and beginnings of electrical activity on the ipsilateral side. Cerebellectomy increases activity on the ipsilateral side. One month after labyrinthectomy there is full electrical activity on both sides, unaffected by the cerebellectomy. (From McCabe and Ryu, 1969, Experiments on vestibular compensation. *Laryngoscope,* **79,** 1728, courtesy of the Editor and Publishers)

CLINICAL APPLICATIONS OF THE BALANCE THEORY

From such a consideration of the balance theory of vestibular function we arrive at two axioms: (1) in vestibular crises of any severity, there will always be labyrinthine nystagmus; (2) if the symptoms last continuously for more than 2 or 3 weeks, the cause is not vestibular.

These axioms can be applied clinically. The first can be helpful if the patient, while dizzy, can be observed by the physician or any instructed person. If, during a significant spell, the patient does not have spontaneous labyrinthine nystagmus, the disease is not vestibular. The physician may not often have the opportunity to observe a spell, because the patient is usually seen between spells. However, the patient's spouse can often be a good observer, once instructed. The physician can do this at the initial visit by pointing out the features of the nystagmus produced by the simple caloric test he performs during his work-up. Some people have become surprisingly astute observers after little instruction. This is an important starting point because it may clearly establish the disease as vestibular or extravestibular early in the diagnostic work-up. If the otolaryngologist is able to establish the nature of the dizziness as non-vestibular, this information is helpful to the referring physician. If he can establish the disease as vestibular, he can proceed to the next important fork in the flow sheet, that of central or peripheral causation.

The second axiom is also helpful in this regard. If, on close questioning, the patient states that his dizziness has been non-episodic and continuous for 2 or 3 months, his disease cannot be vestibular. As previously pointed out, the vestibular system does not function in this manner. There are virtually no clinical exceptions to this axiom.

VESTIBULAR FUNCTION TESTS: WHAT WE CAN LEARN FROM THEM

The goal of vestibular function tests is primarily to decide whether the vestibular disease is end-organ or central in origin. If this can be done with satisfaction, it alone will be a worthy achievement. It is frequently an immense relief to a patient to be told that his complaints are due to end-organ disease and that, whatever follows in the way of symptomatology, his condition will not shorten his life by one day. Even if his disease is not directly treatable, he can at least be assured of eventual relief. If, on the other hand, the disease can be recognized as central, the patient can be put in the hands of the proper specialist until it is diagnosed or until time and the emergence of new symptoms make diagnosis possible. The following vestibular function tests will be discussed in detail below:

(1) Rotation (Barany chair) tests
    Gross difference in the two directions of rotation
    Utility in the child
(2) Electrical tests

(3) Positional tests
     Latency
     Degree of vertigo
     Fatigability
     Direction fixed; direction changing
(4) Caloric tests
     Amount of water at specified temperature
     Hot or cold, or both
     Directional preponderance

Rotation tests

Rotation tests are the oldest of vestibular tests. The major advantage of a rotation test is that cupula deviation can be produced to a precise degree, but this requires sophisticated and expensive equipment. The major disadvantage is that it stimulates both ears at once and gives no laterality information. It should not be considered purely a research test, however, because some clear and useful information can at times be obtained. If, for example, a gross difference (more than 30%) in nystagmus duration is produced by equal spins in the two directions, there either is or has been a significant vestibular incident. This is not specific, but it helps one along the flow sheet to diagnosis. This rotation test can be done simply by putting the patient in any chair that will rotate, fully rotating the patient by hand 10 times in 30 seconds, and then stopping the chair suddenly. After a few minutes, the turns can be repeated in the opposite direction.

Another example of the utility of this test is that it can easily be performed in the young child with apparent severe deafness. Very young children require special audiometric equipment and skills for hearing quantification, such as EEG audiometry, which are available for the most part only in large medical centers. For the rotation test the child can be positioned on the lap of a parent, who holds the head of the child under his own chin so that the heads are on nearly the same axis. The test is then done, and if the child's nystagmus is markedly less than the parent's, particularly if there is little or no nystagmus, it can be accepted that there is severe derangement of the inner ears; immediate and extensive referral is warranted. Although there may appear to be little urgency, experts in education of the deaf are placing hearing aids on children at increasingly earlier ages.

Electrical tests

In this category are only the faradic and galvanic varieties, with the electrode placed over the mastoid cortex to produce a depolarization of the vestibular nerve and precipitate gross movement of the body. The electrical charge necessary to penetrate the skin and temporal bone to the nerve is so large that it is a painful and thus impractical test. Some form of electrical stimulus will be the test of the future, however, for it is precisely quantifiable in terms of strength. Further investigation will undoubtedly give us an electrical stimulus which can be driven without significant pain, much like that used in square-wave testing of the facial nerve.

Positional tests

Positional tests are performed for the detection of positional nystagmus, and can be done with and without visual fixation. With visual fixation, the patient fixates his eyes at a point in each test position, keeping the eyes in cardinal position of gaze. Testing without visual fixation is done with Frenzel glasses or, preferably, by electronystagmography. The usual test positions are upright with head erect, recumbent with left ear down, recumbent with right ear down, and head hanging, with vertex pointed at the floor. Whether the head is moved with the body or the head is moved on the body with neck torsion is not important unless one is seeking to distinguish between gravity-actuated nystagmus and nystagmus produced by vascular embarrassment or from torsion of neck vessels.

The important features of the provoked nystagmus are latency, fatigability, direction changing or direction fixed, degree of vertigo, vegetative symptoms (nausea, cold sweat), and perversion. No latency, or an extremely short one, is indicative of a central lesion; a long latency is indicative of a peripheral lesion. In the latter case, the latency may be as long as 15 or 20 seconds; hence, the position must be held for that period in search of nystagmus. A non-fatigable nystagmus (lasting as long as the position is held) indicates a central lesion; fatigable nystagmus is indicative of a peripheral lesion.

Direction-changing nystagmus is nystagmus which changes in direction from one head position to another or from one examination to another (Aschan type II). Direction-fixed nystagmus is in the same direction regardless of position or time (Aschan type I). Direction-fixed positional nystagmus is virtually always end-organ in origin. The majority (about 80%) of patients with direction-changing nystagmus will also have their lesion in the end-organ but a significantly high percentage of lesions will be central in origin. Therefore, although even a patient with direction-changing nystagmus most likely has an end-organ lesion, this should be a red flag of warning. Such patients deserve redoubled efforts to detect central disease, and their follow-up should be long enough to allow detection of an initially subclinical central process.

The degree of vertigo is high in peripheral lesions and low in central lesions. Thus, a typical patient with a peripheral lesion would be apprehensive of the impending alteration of head position because of the vertigo and would complain of it strongly when it occurred, with the nystagmus, about 5 seconds after the position had been assumed. Within a few seconds, though, both nystagmus and vertigo cease. The converse pattern would indicate a central lesion.

Perverted nystagmus is defined as that which is unexpected in terms of the stimulus. For example, a rotatory nystagmus, upon stimulation of the horizontal semicircular canal, would be perverted. Positional nystagmus of the end-organ variety produces a horizontal-rotatory nystagmus or, less often, a pure rotatory or pure horizontal nystagmus. Thus, a vertical nystagmus on positional testing would be perverted. Perverted nystagmus always means a central lesion.

Postural vertigo is a disease characterized by positional nystagmus. Repeated examinations may be necessary to elicit the nystagmus, but they are essential to a definitive diagnosis. A specific and relatively common form of this disorder is 'benign paroxysmal postural vertigo' (Aschan type III). With the involved ear undermost, after a definite latent period, there appears a rapid labyrinthine nystagmus of brief duration (fatigable), accompanied by intense vertigo. The nystagmus is direction-fixed, and is thought to be of peripheral origin, although this is not certain. Physiologically, it appears to be an otolithic defect, with consequent loss of governing or modulating influence of the otolith organ over the semicircular canals. It is a self-limited disease.

According to a current theory of postural vertigo, cupulolithiasis (Schuknecht), an idiopathically calcified posterior canal cupula is affected by gravity when that ear is placed down, deviating the cupula and producing vertigo and nystagmus. Physiologically, this theory of postural vertigo is untenable, because the system does not work this way. Firstly, once the cupula is deviated, nystagmus results and continues for hours or days until central suppression occurs; in postural vertigo of the end-organ type, the nystagmus with head in place is brief, usually lasting only a few seconds. Adaptation of nystagmic response occurs, but this takes about 40 to 60 seconds and is maximally 40%. Further, the cupula has no 'memory', like polyethylene, to pull it back to zero position with the deviating force still active, for it is a highly damped system. Secondly, existing evidence indicates that the cupula does not move like a fan back and forth, but instead has an anchored tip, the center being the moving portion, much like in a Balinese dancer. In cupulolithiasis, the tip or corner is the calcified portion. Lastly, the posterior canal hair cells are connected only to inferior rectus and superior oblique muscles and are thus able to produce only a vertical nystagmus with an arc component, never a rotatory or horizonal nystagmus (animal experiments). In the human, this is just as true. Patients with a bony fistula of the posterior canal have a vertical nystagmus with an arc. Yet patients with postural vertigo never demonstrate vertical nystagmus; they have a uniformly horizontal or horizontal-rotary or rotary nystagmus. Thus, the theory of cupulolithiasis cannot be accepted on physiologic grounds.

Caloric tests

A variety of caloric tests are used clinically; they differ essentially only in the volume and temperature of water used. The important objectives of caloric testing of the labyrinth are threefold: (1) the stimulus should be sufficient to allow comparison of the two sides; (2) enough stimulus should be provided to evoke all the sequelae of cupula deflection, i.e. nystagmus, vertigo, and vegetative symptoms; (3) a spell is produced for the patient's comparison with his own. Unless these objectives are achieved, much valuable information may be missed. Threshold tests are of limited value because they provide only part of the picture. A suitable screening caloric examination involves irrigation by a stream of 5 ml of ice water over 5 seconds, directed at the posterosuperior quadrant of the tympanic membrane under direct vision. If this does not stimulate each labyrinth to the desired degree, 10 ml of ice water may be used, or, if this is not adequate, 20 ml of ice water, as indicated previously. If ice water does not produce nystagmus or vertigo, that vestibular apparatus is said to be inactive.

The important initial questions to be answered by the caloric test are: (1) does the labyrinth work? (2) does the caloric test qualitatively (not quantitatively) reproduce the patient's spell?

At a minimum, this information should be provided by the caloric test. By following these principles, the discriminating observer can, at times, deduce significant information that may pinpoint the lesion. If enough stimulation is given to evoke all the sequelae of cupular deflection routinely, a missing component may be highly significant. For example, if there is nystagmus and vertigo but no nausea after adequate stimulation, this may indicate a low pontine or medullary lesion with a cut-off of impulses to the dorsal efferent nucleus of X. If there is nystagmus and nausea but no vertigo, this may indicate a midbrain lesion with a cut-off of impulses to higher centers where vertigo is interpreted. If there is vertigo and nausea but no nystagmus, this may indicate a median brain stem lesion with cut-off of impulses to eye muscle nuclei, such as in syringobulbia or multiple sclerosis.

Directional preponderance

Reams of pages have been written about directional preponderance since it was first described four decades ago (Fitzgerald and Hallpike, 1942). In this caloric test, warm and cool water are used in each ear sequentially, usually at 7°C above and 7°C below body temperature, over 30 seconds. All of the right-beating nystagmus time (left cool and right warm) is added and compared with the total left-beating nystagmus time (left warm and right cool). If the right-beating time is greater than the left-beating time, there is a directional preponderance to the right. This is an attractive test because it gives us information in both directions of cupula deviation. It is appropriate as a research test in the quest for new knowledge, but has no place in diagnostic medicine for the following reasons.

We carried out a clinical trial of directional preponderance in 100 subjects with known end-organ or central lesions and 100 'normal' subjects. (It is extremely difficult, if not impossible, to develop a sizable group of normal vestibular subjects because the vestibular system, especially the end-organ and reticular formation, is highly susceptible to common toxins, sedatives, alcohol, barbiturates, and new or old trauma. Traces of toxicity may still be manifest even 48 hours past exposure, yet the subjects are considered normal.) Our results showed a high yield of directional preponderance in the abnormal subjects which was not specific to the lesion, and a high yield of directional preponderance in the normal subjects. What can be said about a diagnostic test which indicates a high incidence of abnormality in normal subjects and normality in abnormal subjects? Moreover, the data in directional preponderance (DP) are based upon the duration of nystagmus, the least valuable and most variable parameter.

We then took our research a step further, using cats as experimental animals. DP was sought in terms of duration of nystagmus as well as other parameters of nystagmus: beat frequency, amplitude, and maximum slow-component speed. The results indicated that directional preponderance of each parameter was present in almost all animals and was due to an order effect, i.e. it was determined by the order in which the ears were irrigated, regardless of the temperature. This is in keeping with a sensory system characterized by adaptation, fatigue, and habituation. A basic weakness of DP testing is the inability to control these variables, and it is therefore worthless as a localizing, or even a general, test of vestibular disease.

Because a waste of time is the only result of DP testing, compared with the caloric response, we advise (and practice) the simple caloric test measured by ENG. After long deliberation over whether to use the single hot or cold stimulation test, we chose the latter, because it is the better discriminator between a paretic canal and one functioning in a normal range. In the lateral canal, kinocilium placement is such that ampullofugal flow (a cold water result) produces a drop in resting discharge, and ampullopetal (a hot water result) a rise in resting discharge.

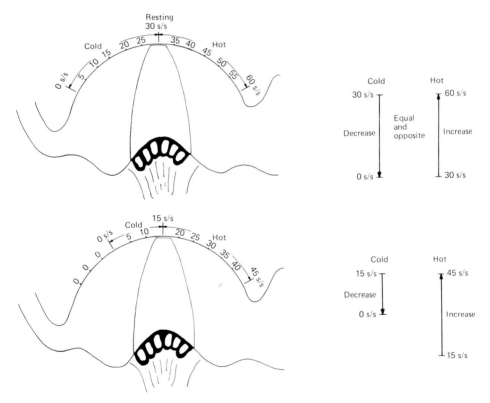

Figure 11.9 Theoretical reasoning behind the adjudged superiority of cold-alone stimulation. The normal crista (*top*) has a resting discharge rate of 30 spikes per second (s/s). Maximum cupula deflection to the right, as produced by hot water or air, increases the resting frequency by 30 s/s, and to the left (cold) decreases it by 30 s/s in a linear manner. If that crista is damaged (*bottom*), reducing its resting frequency to 15 s/s, the cupula will have a shorter range of activity in the direction of the cold deviation, since no greater response can be asked beyond obliteration of the resting frequency. Cold stimulation will be a more discriminating test of abnormality, especially when the stimulus is submaximal. (From McCabe and Ryu, 1979. *Vestibular Physiology in Understanding the Dizzy Patient. Otolaryngology – Head and Neck Surgery,* Rochester, American Academy of Otolaryngology, courtesy of the Editor and Publishers)

Dropping the resting discharge on the damaged side will produce a proportionately greater difference in response on the two sides than raising it, thus making a canal paresis easier to detect (*Figure 11.9*).

We deal with percentage differences of the two sides in determining a significant difference and therefore a canal paresis. Because of the effects of adaptation and the other phenomena, a difference of 20% is not significant; but a 30% difference is arbitrarily significant. On the cold caloric direction of cupula deviation, the system has a narrower range of activity; thus a significant difference of response on the two sides will be easier to detect. A final, if minor, advantage of cold over hot stimulation is that with the use of ice water the clinician has a cheap and readily available stimulus at a constant temperature from one test to the next and one patient to the next.

The simple caloric test

If the physician does only a simple caloric test, without ENG, in order to determine whether the ear works, to make a rough comparison of the relative sensitivity of the two sides, to reproduce a vestibular spell for the patient, and to look for perverted perstimulatory nystagmus, there is another important diagnostic step. Because virtually all dizzy patients fear a spell in a public place, they seldom leave the house alone, and are usually accompanied by a relative. The relative (preferably the spouse or one who lives with the patient) should be invited to note carefully the resultant nystagmus while its features are pointed out by the clinician. He is then instructed to observe the patient's eyes carefully during any future spell for similar movements. The layman, in our experience, can be a remarkably critical observer once trained in this simple way. We have had numerous experiences in which the individual not only described the nystagmus graphically but also gave the direction of nystagmus and the approximate beat frequency. On the other hand, the eyes may be described as non-moving, fixed and staring. In either event, the clinician has clearly passed the first big fork in the flow sheet, i.e. the problem of distinguishing between vestibular and extravestibular disease.

BASIC ELECTRONYSTAGMOGRAPHY

The pioneering research on recording of nystagmus was the work of numerous investigators, and nystagmography has been used by clinicians for evaluating various diseases and by researchers for studying the vestibular system since 1880.

Techniques of evaluating nystagmus

Visual methods

Observations of nystagmus with the naked eye may be augmented by the use of the high-diopter Frenzel (1925) lenses, which make visual fixation by the patient extremely difficult and are a visual aid (as magnifying glasses) to the examiner.

Mechanical methods

A mechanical method was first proposed by Raehlmann (1878) and first used by Hogyes (1899). A metal cup with a writing needle was attached to the cornea, and the first known nystagmogram was recorded on a revolving smoked drum. This method was applied mainly by Buys (1909) and Ohm (1925). Ohm discovered most forms of pathological (eyes open) nystagmus.

Cinematographic method

Attempts to use high-speed movie cameras for recording nystagmus have not been very successful, largely because this method is costly and time-consuming.

Optic method

Mirror images of the cornea are obtained by fixing mirrors to the eyes or reflecting infra-red light from the sclera. Although this method is sensitive enough to record small eye movement, it cannot record rotatory nystagmus.

Photoelectric method

Nykiel and Torok (1963) developed a simplified method for recording nystagmus by using a photoelectric nystagmograph (the sensing device is a photoelectric cell mounted in goggles). This instrument depends on the difference in the reflection of light between the iris and the sclera. It has the advantage of being freely mobile, but it does not eliminate optic fixation and cannot record rotatory nystagmus.

The preceding five methods all have the same limitation: they cannot record nystagmus when the eyes are closed.

Electronystagmography

Electronystagmography (ENG) is a technique for recording nystagmus by means of skin electrodes and an electronic apparatus (*Figure 11.10*). The method was first proposed by Schott (1922) and was applied clinically by Jung (1939). Nystagmus can be recorded by utilizing the corneoretinal potential and its field alterations with eye movements.

Language and function of electronystagmography

The abbreviated term ENG may have any of the following meanings: (1) electronystagmogram, the graphic record of nystagmus obtained by the electro-nystagmograph; (2) electronystagmograph, the apparatus used for the recording of nystagmus; or (3) electronystagmography, the technique used for recording nystagmus by means of skin electrodes and an electronic apparatus.

Principle of ENG

In 1849, Du Bois-Reymond discovered that a potential difference exists between the cornea and the retina (this corneoretinal potential is about 400 to 1100 μV in humans). The cornea was found to be positively charged (*Figure 11.11*). The eyes function as rotating dipoles.

Advantages and disadvantages of ENG

The advantages of ENG are as follows: (1) it allows accurate measurement of nystagmus (velocity of slow and fast components, frequency, amplitude, duration); (2) it can record nystagmus behind closed eyes (latent nystagmus); and (3) a permanent and objective record of nystagmus can be obtained for clinical, research, and medicolegal purposes.

   The following are disadvantages: (1) there is an error due to the polarization of the skin electrode; (2) small eye movements below 1° of angle cannot be recorded because of the poor resolution; (3) a good recording system requires a substantial investment; (4) artifacts make the reading of an ENG difficult for the beginner; and (5) rotatory nystagmus cannot be recorded.

ENG recording system

To record nystagmus by using skin electrodes the following are required: electrodes, preamplifier, amplifiers and recorders.

Type and size of skin electrodes

A small lightweight silver chloride or silver-plated disc (about 15 mm in diameter and 2.5 g in weight) with sodium chloride electro-jelly (ECG paste) is used in clinics and laboratories. In experimental animals, silver needle (26-gauge) electrodes are commonly used, and in some cases silver disc-type electrodes are surgically imbedded for the same purpose.

Placement of electrode

For horizontal nystagmus, electrodes should be placed immediately lateral to the external canthi of the eyes. For vertical nystagmus, electrodes should be placed above the eyebrows and below the lower lids so that they form a vertical line with the pupil of the eye looking straight ahead. The ground electrode (or reference electrode) must be placed on the forehead.

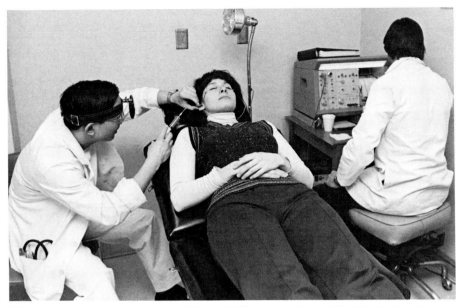

Figure 11.10 ENG room set-up. (From McCabe and Ryu, 1979, *Vestibular Physiology in Understanding the Dizzy Patient. Otolaryngology – Head and Neck Surgery.* Rochester American Academy of Otolaryngology courtesy of the Editor and Publishers)

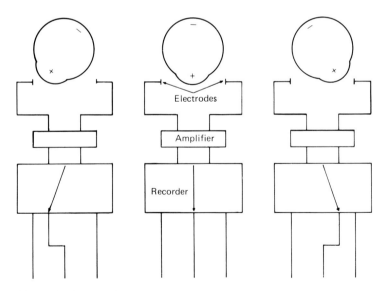

Figure 11.11 Principle of ENG. The eyeball (*top*) is a dipole; its turning changes the electrical field about the forehead. This can be amplified and made to push the pen of a direct writer. (From McCabe and Ryu, 1979, *Vestibular Physiology in Understanding the Dizzy Patient. Otolaryngology – Head and Neck Surgery.* Rochester, American Academy of Otolaryngology, courtesy of the Editor and Publishers)

The baseline of the record

The midline of the recording paper, when the eyes are in the cardinal (forward) position so that the potential difference between two skin electrodes is zero, is called the baseline.

Recording unit

The extremely weak signals which are obtained by the two skin electrodes are first fed into a preamplifier. The preamplified signal is then fed into the input of a power amplifier. The output from the power amplifier drives the recording pen. Various types of ENG recording units are available commercially from several manufacturers. The desirable features of a recording unit are described below.

RESISTOR-CAPACITOR COUPLED VERSUS DIRECT COUPLED SYSTEM
The choice between the direct coupled (DC) system and the resistor-capacitor coupled (AC) system is an individual one, and both systems have advantages and disadvantages. The DC system follows and records the exact movement of the eyes on the recording paper, but the recording pen drifting to its limit of excursion is a problem. With the DC system it is difficult to record the full amplitude of the nystagmic beat unless the pen is reset each time it drifts, or the sensitivity of the recording system is reduced. The AC system with a long time constant, usually 3 to 5 seconds, is popular because this prevents pen drift and allows good nystagmus tracing. However, the AC system with an extremely short time constant does not permit the indication of exact eye movements on the chart.

TIME CONSTANT
The time constant refers to the time it takes a deflected pen to return, on its own, one third of the distance to the baseline.

DIFFERENTIAL PREAMPLIFIER
When dealing with a weak signal, a preamplifier with a differential input capability is preferred over a single-end input unit. A good differential preamplifier has a signal-to-noise ratio of up to 60 dB.

SINGLE OR MULTICHANNEL UNIT
The ENG tracing that is recorded through a single-channel ENG recording unit is known as direct-channel (raw, primary or conventional) tracing. Most parameters of nystagmus (duration, velocity of the slow and fast component, frequency, amplitude) can be computed from this direct-channel tracing. Since the velocity of the slow component of nystagmus is the most accurate indicator of the intensity of nystagmus, its measurement is desirable, and an additional channel (derived, differentiated or velocity channel) is helpful and convenient. The nystagmus is fed into this differentiated channel, which reads out the velocity of the slow component in degrees per second, provided the unit is calibrated. For the purpose of research,

a multichannel ENG recording unit is required, which gives various parameters of nystagmus in various forms (analog or digital) of output.

CALIBRATION
To analyze the electronystagmogram quantitatively, the equipment must be calibrated before each test. This will allow the conversion of pen displacement (cm) to deviation of the eyes in degrees. The simplest method is to place three dots or blinking lights on the wall or the ceiling at a distance of about 2.10 m (7 ft) from the patient. A distance between the dots of about 0.75 m (2.5 ft) will give the eye deviation of 20° (*Figures 11.12 and 11.13*).

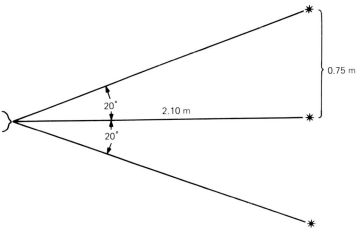

Figure 11.12 Placement of calibration lights. (From McCabe and Ryu, 1979, *Vestibular Physiology in Understanding the Dizzy Patient. Otolaryngology – Head and Neck Surgery.* Rochester, American Academy of Otolaryngology, courtesy of the Editor and Publishers)

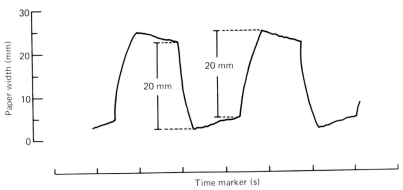

Figure 11.13 Calibration of eye movement: $\dfrac{20° \text{ of eye movement}}{20 \text{ mm of pen deflection}} = 1.0°/\text{mm}.$
(From McCabe and Ryu, 1979, *Vestibular Physiology in Understanding the Dizzy Patient. Otolaryngology – Head and Neck Surgery.* Rochester, American Academy of Otolaryngology, courtesy of the Editor and Publishers)

Other useful information for selecting an ENG recording unit

NECESSARY FEATURES

The following are necessary features of an ENG recording unit: (1) sensitivity (across differential input) of 25 μV input signal, yielding pen deflection of at least 10 mm at maximum gain; (2) a noise level of less than 10 μV peak to peak; (3) gain control with a total range of 80 to 100 dB, and another variable attenuator, with a range of about 10 dB; (4) frequency response, DC to 30 Hz; (5) an input impedance greater than 1.0 MΩ (single-ended) up to 60 Hz, or 0.5 MΩ differentially; (6) a chart containing a full scale of at least 40 mm, and a paper speed of 10 mm/s; and (7) elimination of shock hazard.

DESIRABLE FEATURES

More than one recording channel is desirable. If a DC system is used, the system should have a 'zero suppression'. Variable time constants should be 0.1, 0.3, 0.5, 1, 2, 3 and 5 seconds, and variable paper speed should range from 1 mm/s to 100 mm/s. A rectilinear pen recorder is better than a curvilinear one. A drift of less than 50 V/h and linearity of less than ±2.0% are also desirable.

COMMERCIAL ENG RECORDERS

ENG recorders are available commercially from various manufacturers, including Beckman Instruments, Grass Instruments, Honeywell Instruments, Instrumentation & Control Systems (ICS), Inc., Life-Tech (LT) Instruments, Inc., Texas Medical Instruments and Tracoustics, Inc. Most ECoG, EEG and ECG recorders can be used as an ENG recorder.

Measurements of nystagmus parameters from ENG

Important parameters of nystagmus can be measured from the electronystagmogram.

Duration

The least valuable parameter of nystagmus is total duration (measured in minutes). It is difficult to determine the end-point of nystagmus because near the end of the run gaps occur in the nystagmus, as well as sporadic beats and double beats. One criterion states that the last run of three beats is the end-point.

Total deviation of the slow or fast component

This is expressed in cumulative degrees, radians, or complete eyeball rotations.

Beat frequency

This may also be described in terms of a culmination value, which is defined as the highest best frequency over a period of 10 seconds. This value is variable and heavily affected by drugs, wakefulness, and attentiveness. It is measured in beats per second.

Latency

Measured in seconds, latency is the period between the onset of stimulation and the beginning of a response to the stimulus.

Amplitude

The amplitude of nystagmus can be measured in degrees of radians of each nystagmic beat.

Velocity of the slow (or fast) component

The velocity of the slow component, measured in degrees per second of eyeball speed, most closely correlates with cupular deflection. Maximum velocity is most frequently used as the index of vestibular response. The method of calculating the slow component from the ENG is shown in *Figure 11.14*.

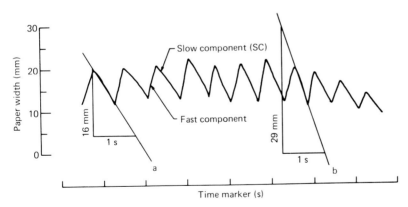

Figure 11.14 Computation of velocity of slow component (SC):
   velocity of SC = slope of SC × calibration;
   velocity of SCa = 16 mm/s × 1.0°/mm = 16°/s;
   velocity of SCb = 29 mm/s × 1.0°/mm = 29°/s.
(From McCabe and Ryu, 1979, *Vestibular Physiology in Understanding the Dizzy Patient. Otolaryngology – Head and Neck Surgery*. Rochester, American Academy of Otolaryngology courtesy of the Editor and Publishers)

CLINICAL ELECTRONYSTAGMOGRAPHY

There is much mythology and witchcraft in the vestibular and ENG literature and a good deal of information that is untrue. This is not the result of any deliberate intention to mislead, but a consequence of both the state of the science at the time and the difficulty inherent in the physiology of a system which is widely integrated into the neuraxis. Two cases in point are directional preponderance and the action of drugs on the vestibular system. We have studied basic mechanisms in our laboratories for almost 20 years as a direct result of the discrepancy which exists between the literature and our own clinical experience. From time to time we have repeated old experiments to determine the experimental error in the original work.

There is a clear and present danger that claims for ENG may become similarly unrealistic. This examination must be kept in perspective; the usefulness of ENG is specific rather than universal and its diagnostic efficacy is limited. The test can be tedious and difficult, and the results misleading if improperly applied. ENG is not like a radiograph or an ECG because it makes no diagnoses (with a few possible exceptions, such as cervical vertigo and cerebellar disease).

The clinician should be satisfied with a positive yield of diagnostic information in no more than 10% to 15% of dizzy patients. One reason for this is that caloric ENG tests only the lateral canal. If the lateral canal is normal, the ENG result will be normal in spite of the presence of a significant lesion in the anterior or posterior canals, the otolith organs or their primary connections, or in any remaining vestibular site. Caloric ENG leaves untested four-fifths of the end-organ neuroepithelium. Another reason for lack of diagnostic yield lies in the construction of the system. It is a system of heavily crossed complex neuron arcs, and virtually every arc has its complement of facilitative and inhibitory arcs. By the time the reflex is read in terms of oculographic response, the lesion is compensated; yet it continues its false message to other arcs which are producing the patient's symptoms.

ENG is in need of refinement, which is dependent on further research. For example, nearly all testing has been related to the vestibulo-ocular arc, although this arc is less likely to produce the patient's symptoms than the vestibulo-spinal tract. There is, however, no clean and efficient way of comparing the right tract with the left, or of quantifying or localizing a lesion in a major brain cord or cord center, or in the end-organs.

It would be a mistake, however, to discard ENG on account of these limitations, because much clear and useful information can be obtained from it. The clinician first needs to set up a protocol of testing which is reasonably efficient in terms of time and patient acceptance and, at the same time, yields maximal information.

Electronystagmography protocol

This ENG protocol is presently in use at the University of Iowa.

(1) Calibrate
(2) Spontaneous nystagmus (eyes open) 60 s. Use alerting
(3) Latent nystagmus (eyes closed) 60 s. Use alerting

(4) Positional nystagmus. Right ear down, left ear down, head hanging – fatigable? Return to sitting between each position. Use alerting
(5) Recalibrate
(6) Intensity response. Back support to 30°. Use alerting
    (a) 5 ml ice water over 5 s. After maximum intensity reached, eyes open and lights on for 10–15 s, then eyes closed
    (b) 10 ml ice water over 10 s. Repeat above
    (c) If no response to 5 and 10 ml, then 20 ml
(7) Monocular tracking, patient cups hand over eye alternately

Steps that provide little or rare information, or are positive only 'when the house is on fire', such as gaze nystagmus and optokinetic nystagmus, are eliminated. The majority of the protocol can be carried out by a trained technician. The caloric irrigation should be done by the clinician himself, not only for medicolegal reasons but also to search for perverted nystagmus, change the alerting mechanism when necessary, and elicit the qualitative similarity of the caloric to the patient's own spell.

Alerting is an extremely important mechanism in ENG testing. Without adequate alerting, it is impossible to validate vestibular fatigue (decruitment) and important signs of central disease, or even to compare the perstimulatory response of the two sides. Signs of alerting failure should be constantly monitored. If the response on the second side tested is less than on the first side, alerting should be switched immediately from mathematical to conversational. It has been shown (Kileny, McCabe and Ryu, 1980) that simply engaging the patient in conversation is the most potent alerting mechanism yet described. It elicits the general arousal reaction (GAR). All parts of the brain are instantly alerted (and reflexes sharpened) as information and commands circuit the brain in preparation for the verbal response which represents the person himself, his own individuality and personality.

Mathematical tasks, on the other hand, can quickly become rote and be relegated to a specific portion of the brain, resulting in diminished alertness. This decline can be detected and the GAR elicited.

Appropriate equipment is necessary for maximal ENG yield. We strongly advocate the use of a two-channel machine, the first channel displaying the raw trace and the second the derived trace (quick-component speed represented by a vertical pen excursion on one side of the baseline, slow on the opposite). The chief reason for this is the frequent need for determining whether or not the wiggles in the raw trace represent nystagmus or simply noise (*Figure 11.15*), as from eyelid twitching. The discovery of latent nystagmus (that present with the lids closed and without stimulation) can be an extremely important yield.

Certain features of the machine should be noted. It should be rugged, and quick repair service should be available. A good machine has good technician acceptance. One should be able to write time-locked comments (e.g. eyes open or closed; start 5 ml; not dizzy) directly on the moving tape. The machine should give a reasonably long time constant, at least 1 second. The case for DC machines is greatly overstated; the AC machine is perfectly adequate, and we prefer it.

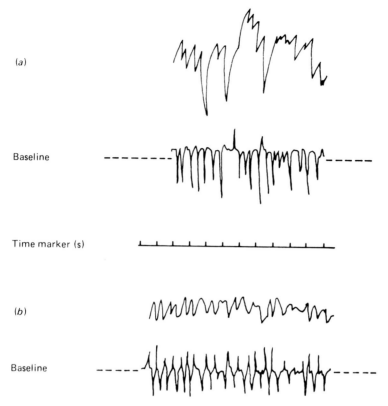

(a)

Baseline

Time marker (s)

(b)

Baseline

Figure 11.15 Use of derived trace to identify presence or absence of nystagmus in raw trace. (*a*) Nystagmus is clearly present because of quicks (below baseline) and slows (above baseline). (*b*) Although raw trace appears to show nystagmus, none is present; derived trace proves absence of quicks and slows. (From McCabe and Ryu, 1979, *Vestibular Physiology in Understanding the Dizzy Patient. Otolaryngology – Head and Neck Surgery*. Rochester, American Academy of Otolaryngology, courtesy of the Editor and Publishers)

Finally, the clinician should analyze the tape himself and not be content with reading a report. It is his or her responsibility to examine the data, just as it is the cardiologist's responsibility (and not the technician's) to interpret the ECG trace.

ENG interpretation

The following is a minimal listing of points of interpretation which should be sought, and the protocol for eliciting them.

Latent nystagmus

Note direction and speed. Refer to derived trace for proof of nystagmus and not noise.

Positional nystagmus

Note direction, latency, fatigability, degree of vertigo, and direction-fixed and direction-changing characteristics.

Comparison of sensitivity of the two sides

Note maximum speeds of slow component. Canal paresis is present if one side is weaker by 30% or more.

The hyperexcitable (hyperirritable) labyrinth

We do not believe the hyperirritable labyrinth exists in clinical neurology, with the possible exception of the destructive phase of acute suppurative labyrinthitis, when there is massive ongoing depolarization during the first 60 to 100 min, with waxing and waning nystagmus to the involved ear. Calorization of the involved ear results in flashes of incredibly fast nystagmus, too fast for measurement by our standard low-frequency response machines. (This is a specific disease, however, not requiring ENG for diagnosis but primarily a competent clinical otolaryngologist.) The condition raises the question, 'What is the upper limit of slow-component speed for the normal system?' We do not know, but we have seen speeds in excess of 80 degrees per second in normal subjects! Thus, we do not believe the hyperexcitable labyrinth to be an entity, but have included it here for comment.

Cervical nystagmus elicitation

When cervical vertigo is suspected (as in whiplash injury, head and neck trauma, or symptoms of neck torsion), special maneuvers should be included in the protocol to produce the vertigo and record bursts of nystagmus during symptoms. Only in this way can cervical vertigo be diagnosed with certainty, unless the nystagmus is spontaneous (present with eyes open) and thus visible. These maneuvers should include head-on-neck positions, which the patient avoids in order to prevent symptoms. Another helpful maneuver is 'lifting the head without really lifting it', sometimes called the McCabe maneuver. The patient, supine with leads in place, is instructed to start lifting the head off the table without actually lifting it from the table any more than to allow a piece of paper to slide from under the head. Thus, all the neck muscles, particularly the deep muscles, are tensed without any actual arc or position movement of the head. A burst of three or more beats is diagnostic. It may be repeatable or non-repeatable, thus requiring repeated testing (more than one visit); absence of nystagmus on any one test does not rule out the diagnosis.

Central versus peripheral signs

Here, ENG has one of its most useful applications. With determination of central or peripheral locus, the second big fork in the flow sheet is passed. A number of ENG features are important, and the protocol should be set up to elicit them.

DIRECTION-CHANGING NYSTAGMUS ON POSITIONAL TESTING

This is one of the poorer signs, since only about 20% of patients with central disease have it. When present, however, it should be a 'red flag of warning'.

CALIBRATION OVERSHOOT

ENG calibration is the initial step in the protocol. Basically, this seeks to match a certain number of degrees of eyeball arc with the same number of millimeters of pen trace on the machine. The result on the tape is a series of square waves. Calibration overshoot (of the eye track) is recognized by the appearance of spikes on the corners of the square waves (*Figure 11.16*). There is an 83% correlation

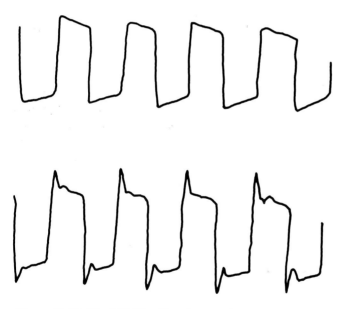

Figure 11.16 (*Top*) ENG calibration result on the tape is a series of square waves (without overshoo' ʝ. (*Bottom*) Calibration overshoot is seen as spikes on the corners of the square waves. Overshoot must occur in more than 50% of the square waves to be significant

between calibration overshoot and cerebellar disease (Haring and Simmons, 1973), an extremely high correlation for ENG. It is a manifestation of ocular dysmetria. Cerebellar disease is, of course, not a diagnosis to the neurologist (cerebellar medulloblastoma, for example, would be), but to the neurotologist it is a diagnosis. For a positive test, spikes on at least 50% of the square waves are required. This is a particularly attractive test, because it adds no time to the ENG.

PENDULUM TRACKING

The pendulum should have a frequency of 0.5 Hz at an amplitude of 15° to 20° (Corvera, Torres-Courtney and Lopez-Rio, 1973). It must be performed monocularly, with one eye covered with a card (rather than closed voluntarily) to avoid lid artifact. It is necessary to test one eye at a time, because the abnormal eye tracks normally with the good eye by tandem harness effect. It is another test for ocular dysmetria and indicates brain stem or cerebellar disease centrally, or end-organ asymmetry peripherally.

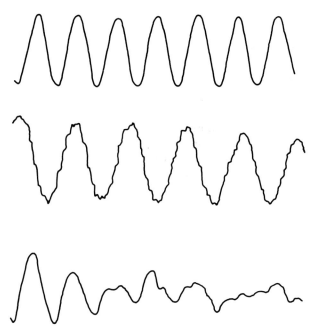

Figure 11.17 Pendulum tracking. (*Top*) Normal, smooth sine wave; (*center*) superimposed wiggly trace, indicating end-organ disease; (*bottom*) loss of recognizable sine wave, indicating CNS disease. (From McCabe and Ryu, 1979, *Vestibular Physiology in Understanding the Dizzy Patient. Otolaryngology – Head and Neck Surgery*. Rochester, American Academy of Otolaryngology, courtesy of the Editor and Publishers)

Three types of tracking are identifiable (*Figure 11.17*): (1) a smooth, regular sine wave which is the normal trace but is also compatible with end-organ disease; (2) a sine wave with superimposed wiggly trace, which is seen only with end-organ disease in the absence of a visual defect, such as refraction error; and (3) gross break-up of the sine wave so that it is virtually undiscernible, which indicates central disease.

LOSS OF FIXATION SUPPRESSION OF CALORIC NYSTAGMUS

This is sometimes referred to as a positive ocular fixation index. Normally, when the eyes are opened in a lighted room during the nystagmus run, the amplitude of nystagmus and the speed of the slow component are significantly and visibly diminished. This maneuver is carried out after the speed of the slow component has reached its maximum. If there is no significant change, and particularly when amplitude and the speed of the slow component increase compared with that of the closed eye, central disease is present. The absence of fixation suppression does not rule out a central lesion; the lesion must be in the vestibulo-ocular arc to be positive. When present, however, it is a significant sign. We need clinical research in this area to determine whether testing of one eye at a time gives greater yield than binocular testing. Another attractive feature of this test is that it adds no time to the ENG.

DECRUITMENT (CALORIC PERSTIMULATORY FATIGUE)
This test elicits neuronal arc fatigue by comparing the effect of a weak stimulus (5 ml ice water caloric) with that of a stronger (10 ml ice water) stimulus. The stronger stimulus should elicit as fast a maximal slow-component speed or a faster one. If it is significantly less, fatigue is present, and this is a sign of central disease (Torok, 1975). The clinician should be particularly careful to note loss of alertness and should reinforce this by conversation, looking for maximum slow-component speed to break through. This test is usually done near the end of the ENG when the patient is tired. If fatigue is observed, the drug history should be retaken, since these agents are the most common offenders. Virtually all vestibular drugs act centrally.

Restatement on fatigue

Confusion may result from the use of the term 'fatigue' to describe phenomena of both peripheral and central responses. Unfortunately, the term has crept into the literature to typify both these responses, but they must be kept distinct. Fatigue in positional nystagmus is indicative of end-organ disease. 'Adaptation' is a better term because it is closer to that mechanism, although other factors are operative as well (adaptation is only a reducer and not an eliminator). Fatigue in serially increasing caloric response is indicative of central disease and is due to early overload of a neuron arc.

PATHOPHYSIOLOGY OF DISEASES CAUSING VERTIGO

Ménière's disease

Current best opinion and cumulative clinical and experimental evidence all suggest that the fundamental defect in Ménière's disease is an endolymphatic hypertension due to deficient absorption and drainage of endolymph, producing a hydropic dilatation of the endolymphatic compartment. It has its analog in many other body organs producing a similar type of disease: hydrocephalus, hydramnios, glaucoma, lymphedema, hydrocele, hydronephrosis, gall bladder hydrops.

Membrane rupture is not uncommon in otology and, in the oval and round windows, is due to either focal membrane erosion (as by a prosthesis) or abnormal perilymphatic fluid pressures or middle ear pressures. In Ménière's disease, abnormal endolymphatic fluid pressure causes ruptures, usually in Reissner's membrane, the thinnest of the inner ear membranes (having no connective tissue layer). Inner ear fluids then mix, producing an unfavorable ionic environment for the sensory cell transducers, and massive depolarization occurs; this leads to the typical vestibular seizure and flattening of hearing acuity. Reissner's membrane repairs itself, ionic equilibrium is restored, and the spell ceases. Many sensory cells are injured and recover, but some are killed so that after a number of spells the hearing and vestibular function suffer progressively in time. Membrane ruptures which occur solely in the pars superior result in Ménière's disease without deafness, but this is relatively uncommon, accounting for less than 5% of cases. Pars inferior ruptures can occur repeatedly low in the cochlea without significant diffusion of perilymph into the pars superior; Ménière's disease without vertigo is the result.

The numerous operations for Ménière's disease can be evaluated with respect to the degree to which they consistently perform their mission; for example, endolymphatic sac drainage operations are effective if the sites do not later close with fibrosis; endolymphatic decompression operations produce the desired effect where the sac is large enough and supple enough to effect decompression; and efficacious vestibular nerve sections produce secretomotor denervation of the dark cells on the slopes of the cristae, diminishing endolymph production.

The high effectiveness of conservative treatment for Ménière's disease (1000 mg sodium diet plus high doses of diazide diuretics) appears to be a direct result of the lowered volume of inner ear fluid in the entire extracellular fluid compartment.

The goals of therapy in the modern otological era are no longer merely to stop the major spells, but also to stabilize or improve hearing. An ear in which hearing continues to deteriorate must be considered a treatment failure. Today we rarely resort to totally destructive operations for that reason, and for the reason that especially those of us involved in the cochlear implant program are deeply impressed by how precious even a little hearing is.

The result of medical therapy in our hands is long-term resolution of all major spells in 75% of patients. However, in only 42% of patients is stabilization or improvement of hearing achieved. Thus, 58% are failures in terms of the goals of treatment. The majority of patients not responding to medical treatment later undergo an operative procedure. Not all patients, however, receive an operation for failure of control of spells, because some are quite content to be relieved of all but one major spell per year. And not all patients with deteriorating hearing receive an operation for stabilization or improvement of hearing, because these results cannot be guaranteed. The first operation chosen is usually an endolymphatic shunt into the mastoid chamber, which results in stabilization or improvement in 62% of patients. In the shunt group then, 38% continue to have spells and/or deterioration of hearing. Shunt failures are treated by a middle fossa vestibular nerve section. Translabyrinthine vestibular nerve sections are not performed unless there is no hearing in that ear. Nerve section results in stabilization or improvement of hearing in 20% of these patients. The remaining 80% continue to have deterioration of hearing. It is of interest that in the latter group approximately one-third of patients have late deterioration of hearing, after an initial stabilization or improvement. This is evidence that the nerve section does nothing to reverse the basic nature of the disease, which continues to exist in the cochlea. All patients in this group have complete control of spells of vertigo.

Postural vertigo

Peripheral postural vertigo, which accounts for about 90% of cases, is best explained by a focal microscopic loss of otolithic macular neuroepithelium resulting from either a neurovirus or a microstroke. Most otolithic neuroepithelium is in a state of resting discharge activity (tonic neuron activity) or is silent (kinetic neuron activity) in the upright head position. With a change of head position from the upright, selective areas of maculae specific to that position are stimulated orthogonally on the two sides, and equal but opposite neuronal discharges volley into the vestibular nuclei. When the head position is assumed, after the lesion-involving evocation of an area now damaged, this end-organ cannot produce its equal and opposite fund of discharges, and asymmetry and symptoms (including nystagmus) result. Immediately after the head is moved out of that position, the asymmetry subsides and symptoms cease. Resolution is through the mechanism of central compensation. In time, usually 4 to 5 months, the equivalent of the input from the denervated area of macula is built up in that small volume of vestibular nucleus discharged upon, and equilibration is restored in terms of electrical activity. When that happens, asymmetries no longer occur. The stimulus to this regeneration of electrical activity in the nucleus is the spell, which explains efficacy of labyrinthine exercises in this disease. The greater the frequency of spells, the sooner this equivalency is built up in the involved nucleus and the shorter the duration of the symptoms.

Mention should be made here of cupulolithiasis, which cannot be the cause of postural vertigo, because this would be a totally unphysiological process. Firstly, the neurons of the posterior crista drive the superior oblique and inferior rectus extraocular muscles. Thus, when the posterior canal cupula is deviated, vertical nystagmus with a slight rotatory quality results. This has been demonstrated repeatedly by electrical stimulation of the singular nerve experimentally. In patients with postural vertigo, horizontal or horizontal-rotatory rather than vertical nystagmus is seen. Secondly, the nystagmus in postural vertigo is characterized by a definite period of latency and is of quite brief duration. It is physiological, however, for nystagmus to begin immediately when the cupula is deviated, and to continue for as long as the cupula is deviated. It has been demonstrated experimentally that the cupula has no 'spring-back' capacity of its own. 'Adaptation' cannot be the reason for the brevity of the nystagmus; as long as the cupula is deviated, nystagmus continues for hours to days and is not a peripheral but a central extinction phenomenon. Cupulolithiasis cannot account for the pathophysiology of postural vertigo, because the system simply does not work this way.

Viral labyrinthitis (vestibular neuronitis)

The pathophysiology of this disease remains enigmatic because we have no disease of temporal bones to demonstrate where the damage lies. We believe it to be viral for two reasons: (1) there is frequently a history of viral upper respiratory infection shortly before onset of the disease; (2) it has been reported several times in epidemic form at armed forces bases. The symptoms are classic and consist of a single severe vestibular crisis lasting about 1 week, with gradual resolution of symptoms and without auditory involvement. Symptoms include 3° of horizontal nystagmus to the uninvolved side, nausea and vomiting. Calorization of the affected ear results in no change in the nystagmus; thus, there is a canal paralysis. Calorization of the opposite ear with cold water stops the nystagmus temporarily. Approximately two-thirds of the ears recover and normal reflexes return; the remainder lose function permanently. In the latter, symptoms of asymmetry (motion intolerance, postural vertigo) may last for weeks or months until central compensation is complete. Treatment is with diazepam for the acute spell, and labyrinthine exercises for residual symptoms persisting for more than 2 weeks.

Toxic labyrinthitis

Labyrinthitis due to lead, arsenic, zinc, metal-fume fever or quinine rarely occurs today. Since credence in the 'focus of infection' theory of disease has waned, this diagnosis is seldom made. The clearest examples of toxic labyrinthitis are the direct toxic effects of ototropic antibiotics, of which we have a host today. Among these are kanamycin, viomycin, neomycin, colistin, streptomycin, and dihydrostreptomycin. Apparently, these drugs directly affect the hair cell. Patients who need ototoxic antibiotics are those who are extremely ill or in a life-threatening situation and will not respond to non-toxic antibiotics. In any other circumstances these antibiotics are not indicated, and the otolaryngologist should take the lead in the promulgation of this tenet. If hearing does not drop concomitantly with vestibular loss, toxic labyrinthitis may not be discovered until the patient ambulates or attempts to ambulate, since the labyrinthitis is bilaterally symmetric and auto-cancelling in effect, until the need for active labyrinths is called forth by stimulation.

Toxic labyrinthitis is generally dose-related, and within the safe prescribed limits of dosage of the antibiotic there is usually only minimal loss of vestibular sensitivity and no frank toxic labyrinthitis. Another form of toxic labyrinthitis, however, is not dose-related but appears to be more of an antigen–antibody reaction or anaphylactic response. With dosages which are ordinarily within safe limits, both vestibular labyrinths may be rendered inactive. I have seen 5 patients with normal thermal vestibulograms, who after receiving 5–9 g (doses of 1 g/day) of streptomycin sulfate, had each labyrinth rendered totally inactive to a 20 ml ice water caloric test.

Acute suppurative labyrinthitis

This disease is more commonly a sequela of chronic than acute suppurative mastoiditis. The symptoms are always sudden in onset, preceded only by a chronic draining ear. The patient is prostrated with a vestibular crisis which includes marked vertigo, nystagmus, nausea and vomiting. The hearing in the ear is not immediately destroyed but may be greatly reduced. The nystagmus is toward the infected ear for the first 1 to 3 hours. A diminution or temporary cessation of the nystagmus then occurs, whereupon it begins to beat to the opposite, or normal, ear. At this time the hearing in the ear is totally erased, the vestibular reaction is totally absent, and the ear is said to be 'dead'. The situation is urgent, and labyrinthectomy must be performed to prevent spread to the meninges. This operation is carried out usually after a brief period of intensive antibiotic therapy. The nystagmus continues to beat to the opposite ear postoperatively until central compensation has occurred, usually in a matter of 1 to 2 weeks.

Serous labyrinthitis

This is a sterile form of labyrinthitis, the most common causes of which are trauma and adjacent infection. Nystagmus may be present to either ear, although it is usually to the opposite ear. The nystagmus lasts for several hours or, at most, several days, and may be constant. Positional changes may intensify or diminish the nystagmus. Hearing may be impaired, but not severely depressed. The auditory manifestations of hair cell irritation may be present. Sensitivity to vestibular tests may be diminished in the involved ear, but not totally lost. The lesion of serous labyrinthitis is usually entirely reversible, although there may be some loss of threshold sensitivity in the vestibular compartment. Classic examples of serous labyrinthitis are those states of vestibular irritation following fenestration and stapedectomy. It may also be an accompaniment of acute suppurative otitis media, presumably a consequence of the diffusion of bacterial products through the round window membrane, without passage of the bacteria.

Circumscribed labyrinthitis

By definition, this condition obtains when there is a positive fistula test in the presence of chronic suppurative otitis media and mastoiditis. On compression of air in the external auditory canal, there is a deviation of the eyes to the opposite side; on rarefaction of air in the canal, deviation of the eyes toward the affected ear occurs. Suppurative osteitis has occurred up to the endosteum of the membranous labyrinth but not invading the labyrinth. The positive fistula test results from compression of the endosteum of the lateral semicircular canal against the lateral semicircular duct, which forces endolymph in both an anterior and a posterior direction from the point of compression. The anteriorly displaced endolymph causes cupula deflection toward the utricle. Anterior cupular deflection in the lateral canal rotates the eyes in the same direction as the cupula, away from the ear. The variety of vertigo the patient experiences during the disease is low-grade, tends to come in waves, and disappears after a few seconds or minutes. Nausea is inconsequential or absent, and there are no vertiginous spells during crisis. The

crisis. The hearing is depressed, but the loss is primarily conductive and due to the chronic infection. The patient may volunteer that he dares not put his finger in his ear because this will knock him sideways. This condition constitutes another otological urgency, for the infection must be eliminated before it invades the labyrinth and results in acute suppurative labyrinthitis, which will kill the ear.

Perilabyrinthitis

This condition may develop after mastoidectomy in a healing cavity. The primary symptoms are motion intolerance and usually a partial sensorineural deafness of the cochlear type. The motion intolerance is aptly described as the 'supermarket syndrome', wherein the patient cannot tolerate looking back and forth among aisles and up and down shelves because of the considerable head motion required. The syndrome results in vegetative symptoms (nausea, pallor, cold sweat), marked unsteadiness and a feeling of impending disaster.

In perilabyrinthitis, infection of the mastoidectomy wound results in acutely infected bone of the labyrinth capsule, without bone destruction to the endosteum. The fistula test is therefore negative. There may be infected granulation tissue growing on bone. The symptoms are produced by inflammatory irritation of the labyrinth causing overreaction of normal vestibular reflexes or, possibly, blunting of the otolith system on responses. Caloric responses of the canals are retained. The lesion is reversible, and responds to specific systemic antibiotics (since this is an acute osteitis) and to intensive cavity care. Depending on the original operation (i.e. 'canal-up' procedure or endaural approach), the postauricular incision is opened or a new incision is made which is left open for intensive cavity care, and closed after the infection has subsided. The hearing loss is generally reversible. A revision mastoidectomy may be necessary, but this should not be the case if the original operation has been adequately performed. As in virtually all labyrinthine disorders, diazepam is most helpful in controlling acute symptoms during the recovery phase.

Cervical vertigo

This relatively common disorder is usually caused by whiplash injury to the cervical spine or by head on neck trauma. Certain positions of the head on neck, particularly neck extension and neck torsion, will produce acute vertigo and nystagmus, although the nystagmus is variable in its presence, even on ENG. When the nystagmus is visible or recordable, it is diagnostic. Motion intolerance is invariable and may prevent the patient from performing his gainful occupation. Chronic posterior neck pain, occipital headache, or both, are common. Deep neck muscle tenderness is present. Cervical vertigo is seen predominantly in females, possibly because of their lesser mass of neck musculature stabilizing the neck against a severe sudden excursion of the head. Patients with cervical vertigo are frequently labelled neurotic because of the paucity of physical findings, the bitter complaint of symptoms, and the usual presence of impending litigation.

The disease has a definite experimental basis, however. Cervical vertigo can be produced in the experimental animal by blocking the dorsal cervical nerve roots with local anesthesia on one side. Nystagmus, ataxia, and circling movements result, lasting for several hours. The precise lesion in cervical vertigo is not known and may be in neck musculature, sensory nerves of the neck, cervical vertebral joints, or the cervical spinal cord. Fibrosis is apparently an important element of the disease. Indeed, a feature which may lead the clinician away from the diagnosis is the usual delay of 2–4 weeks between the injury and the emergence of symptoms. This interval strongly suggests fibrosis producing distortion of anatomic structures. The basic process in the production of symptoms is most likely that abnormal volleys of impulses reach the vestibular nuclei via spinovestibular tracts.

The treatment is conservative, consisting of a soft cervical collar (worn during all upright hours) to take the weight of the head off the neck, and prolonged diazepam 5 to 39 mg daily. The longer the delay in treatment, the less the response to treatment will be, so that after 6 months only a 50% reduction in symptoms can be expected. In assessing results it is important to keep a log of which tasks the patient could not perform before treatment and becomes able to perform during treatment, because patients tend to complain just as bitterly about residual symptoms as about pretreatment symptoms. Psychotherapy has no demonstrable effect on symptoms or treatment outcome.

Vertigo from vascular loops

This is a definite disease entity which the author has diagnosed and treated in 6 patients to date. The vascular loop syndrome is difficult to diagnose because no tests are specific for it. Patients present with the exact clinical picture of unilateral Ménière's disease, with typical episodic seizures of vertigo, and auditory test results are compatible with Ménière's disease. In addition, the vascular loop patient has considerably more motion intolerance than the Ménière's patient such that they cannot ride a bicycle, or travel in a boat, or even a car, comfortably. The significant feature in distinguishing this syndrome from Ménière's disease is its total failure to respond to therapy for Ménière's disease. Medical therapy, shunt surgery, and even destructive labyrinthotomy or labyrinthectomy fail to control it. The only treatment which alleviates the symptoms permanently is middle fossa resection of the vestibular nerve at the point of impingement of the vascular loop. At operation, a loop of the anterior inferior cerebellar artery (or a branch from it) is found extending into the medial half of the internal auditory canal, visibly impinging upon and indenting the vestibular nerve. In 1 of 6 patients a double loop was found, with the vestibular nerve passing between. In the segment between the loops the nerve was flattened to about one-third of its diameter between the loops.

It is possible that the late generation, high resolution CT scanners could show the vascular loop with air studies.

References

Buys, E. (1909) De la nystagmographie clinique. *Monatsschrift für Ohrenheilkunde*, **43**, 801

Corvera, J., Torres-Courtney, G. and Lopez-Rio, G. (1973) The neurotological significance of alterations of pursuit eye movement and the pendular eye tracing test. *Annals of Otology, Rhinology and Laryngology*, **82**, 855

Du Bois-Reymond, E. (1849) Untersuchungen über thieriscge Elektrizität. Berlin: G. Reimer, **2**, 256

Fitzgerald, G. and Hallpike, C. S. (1942) Studies in human vestibular function. I. Observation of the directional preponderance (Nystagmusbereitschaft) of caloric nystagmus resulting from cerebral lesion. *Brain*, **65**, 115

Frenzel, H. (1925) Nystagmus beobachtung mit einer 'Leuchtbrille'. *Klinische Wochenschrift*, **4**, 138

Haring, R. D. and Simmons, B. F. (1973) Cerebellar defects detectable by electronystagmography calibration. *Archives of Otolaryngology*, **98**, 14–17

Hogyes, A. (1899) Neuere experimentelle Beiträge zur Kenntnis der Reflexbeziehungen zwischen Ohr und Auge, *Mathematikai es terme szettudo man, ertezito*

Jung, R. (1939) Eine elektrische Methode zur mehrfachen Registrierung von Augenbewegungen und Nystagmus. *Klinische Wochenschrift*, **1**, 21

Kileny, P., McCabe, B. F. and Ryu, J. H. (1980) Effects of attention requiring tasks on vestibular nystagmus. *Annals of Otology, Rhinology and Laryngology*, **89**, 9

McCabe, B. F. (1973) Summary of neurotology symposium on vestibular diagnosis. *Annals of Otology, Rhinology and Laryngology*, **82**, 869

Nykiel, F. and Torok, N. (1963) A simplified nystagmograph. *Annals of Otology, Rhinology and Laryngology*, **72**, 647

Ohm, J. (1925) Ein neuer Nystagmograph. *Klinische Wochenschrift*, **4**, 1286

Raehlmann, E. (1878) Über den Nystagmus und seine Aetiologie. *Archiv für Ophthalmologie*, **24**, 237

Schott, E. (1922) Über die Registrierung des Nystagmus und anderer Augenbewegungen vermittels des Saitengalvanometers. *Deutsches Archiv für klinische Medizin*, **140**, 79

Torok, N. (1975) Posterior fossa lesions and vestibular decruitment. In *Proceedings of the Fifth Extraordinary Meeting of the Barany Society*, edited by M. Merimoto, p. 196. *International Journal of Equilibrium Research* (*Kyoto*)

12
Fluctuant hearing loss
D. Plester

Fluctuant hearing loss is a common clinical complaint, often accompanied by the sensation of fullness in the ear, roaring tinnitus and vertigo. With fluctuant hearing, the hearing threshold varies between two extremes, the normal or reduced stable hearing component, and the superimposed fluctuant reversible component.

The three following types of fluctuant hearing loss have to be distinguished:

(1) fluctuant conductive hearing loss
(2) fluctuant sensory (cochlear) hearing loss
(3) fluctuant neural (retrocochlear) hearing loss

FLUCTUANT CONDUCTIVE HEARING LOSS

Serous otitis media

Serous otitis media is certainly the most frequently encountered cause of fluctuant conductive hearing loss of the middle ear type. The conductive component of the hearing loss is due to the fluid in the middle ear. There is almost always a sensorineural component in the high frequency range as well (Arnold and Ganzer, 1980; Münker, 1980). Diffusion of oxygen through the round window membrane into the inner ear, which is possible in normal healthy ears, might not be possible in ears with serous otitis media and this has been quoted to explain the sensorineural hearing loss in serous otitis media. Investigations in our department by Hlobil (1979) have shown that the temporary threshold shift following sound exposure is smaller in patients with serous otitis media than in normal individuals, demonstrating that there is no disturbance of inner ear metabolism.

Because the decreased bone conduction threshold improves to a normal threshold immediately after removal of the serous or mucous fluid from the middle ear, the sensorineural component is only a 'pseudoperceptive' deafness (Huizing, 1964), comparable with the 'Carhart notch' in otosclerosis, and is due to the 'mass-loading' effect of the fluid on the round window membrane.

216

Otomandibular syndrome

This syndrome is not well known in otology. The main complaints are of pain in and around the ear, fullness in the ear, a fluctuant hearing loss, tinnitus and a sensation of unsteadiness. In order to understand the close relationship between the ear and mandible we have to refresh our embryological knowledge. In the very early stages of development the same branchial arch gives rise to the formation of the tensor tympani as well as to the medial pterygoid muscle. Both are innervated by the mandibular branch of the trigeminal nerve. The third muscle, innervated by the mandibular branch of the fifth cranial nerve, is the tensor veli palatini, which is not related to mastication but to Eustachian tube function, that is, the opening of the Eustachian tube. When dysfunction of the masticatory apparatus has been present for any length of time, several masticatory muscles become spastic. The same mechanism which produces the spasm of the masticatory apparatus influences the tensor tympani and tensor veli palatini muscles as well. Their dysfunction explains the symptomatology described by Klockhoff and Westerberg (1973) as the 'tonic tensor tympani phenomenon'.

Klockhoff (1976) wrote 'fifteen patients, who were referred for hearing dysfunction and who exhibited the 'tonic tensor phenomenon', were interviewed about other complaints. Thirteen were found to be suffering from tension headaches, one from tension headaches and otalgia, and one from otalgia only. In addition to headache many patients complained of fullness in the ear, abnormalities of sound perception and dizziness. For this combination of symptoms, the 'tensor tympani syndrome' might be an adequate term. The previous diagnosis in many cases was atypical Ménière's disease or simply neurosis'.

Some authors have shown that tonic contraction of the tensor tympani muscle causes changes in impedance and in pure tone audiometry, such as a slight conductive loss in the low frequencies. The conductive loss is explained by tubal or tensor tympani dysfunction but there is frequently some influence on the inner ear function as well, resulting in a fluctuant sensorineural hearing loss.

Patients with otomandibular problems usually have psychological problems, which they express by tensing their muscles of mastication, by clenching or by grinding their teeth. Besides psychological factors severe enough to necessitate a psychological evaluation, malocclusion or dental malfunction are very often involved in this problem. The pain, tinnitus and hearing loss are usually found in one ear only. The investigation of the temporomandibular joint during movements of the mandible and the palpation of the medial and lateral pterygoid muscles will give some information about their function.

Approximately half of our patients presenting with unexplained ear symptoms of the above-mentioned nature showed a significant improvement, or became symptom-free, after adequate specific treatment in our dental department.

FLUCTUANT SENSORY (COCHLEAR) HEARING LOSS

Round window fistula

Patients with round window fistulae generally present with a severe sensorineural hearing loss of sudden onset, vertigo and roaring tinnitus. The aetiology is not clear in every case, but barotrauma or suddenly increased cerebrospinal fluid pressure, which often follows physical strain, diving, etc., are postulated to lead to the rupture of the round and/or oval windows. Fluctuant hearing loss of sudden onset may be the only sign. Patients with a sudden sensorineural hearing loss and a suggestive history of physical stress who show no improvement after medical treatment of about 10 days should probably have a surgical exploration. Tympanoscopy is considered as a diagnostic procedure in patients with a clinically suspected rupture of the labyrinthine windows. Fistulae can only be confirmed and treated by this intervention.

Oval window fistula

Fistulae of the oval window are less common after pressure changes in the middle or inner ear, but they are sometimes seen after stapedectomy, depending on the surgical technique employed. The symptomatology is similar to that of rupture of the round window membrane. In our experience the vestibular symptoms are more pronounced, the hearing loss is not so severe and it is often of a combined sensorineural/conductive type. The fluctuant hearing loss is mostly due to fluctuations in the bone conduction threshold. The conductive hearing loss is rather stable. The quality of the tinnitus is the same in patients with round or oval window membrane ruptures.

Ménière's disease

The most important disease of the inner ear causing fluctuant hearing loss, vertigo and tinnitus is Ménière's disease. The sudden onset of the disabling, spinning vertigo with vomiting, roaring and in some cases pulsating tinnitus, together with hearing loss and the sensation of fullness or pressure in the ear, is a dramatic event for the patient and for the inexperienced physician. Patients with a classical Ménière's attack are sometimes admitted to hospital with the diagnosis of a cerebrovascular accident or an acute gastrointestinal disorder.

Anatomy, histopathology and pathophysiology

Anatomical, histological and biochemical studies performed over the last two decades have extended our knowledge about the pathophysiology of this peculiar disease but little is known about its aetiology.

Two factors seem to predispose to the development of the disease: the anatomy of the sac and perisaccular fibrosis; a trigger mechanism then leads to the clinically manifested disease.

Planimetric measurements of the pneumatization of the temporal bone have revealed that the extent of pneumatization is significantly reduced in patients with Ménière's disease, compared with normal individuals (Pirker, 1976). However, there is no significant difference in the degree of pneumatization between the diseased and the normal ear in the same patient with Ménière's disease. We are not sure whether these findings are in any way related to the special anatomical position of the endolymphatic sac in Ménière's disease.

In most papers dealing with operations on the endolymphatic sac, the identification of the structure is described as difficult, and in 5–10 % of cases it may be impossible. In our experience the situation of the sac in Ménière's disease is slightly anterior, medial and inferior to the classically described anatomical position. This clinical observation in patients with Ménière's disease, which I described in 1972, and which was later confirmed by Arenberg *et al.* (1977) in an extensive radiological and clinical study, indicates that the abnormal position of the sac might be a predisposing factor in this disease. A small dimple in the tabula interna of the posterior fossa is also a valuable landmark when looking for the sac. Other typical findings, apart from the anomalous position, are that the sac is small and whitish with perisaccular fibrosis, that it is poorly vascularized and that there are multiple intrasaccular adhesions. In comparison with a normal sac there is almost no lumen and the sac can be described as 'atelectatic'.

Shambaugh (1975) thinks a viral infection in childhood that has spread into the inner ear, with the virus particles then being transported into the sac by a flow of endolymph, might be the cause of these rather marked changes. The labyrinth can still maintain hydrostatic equilibrium through its resorbing cells in other areas until adulthood, when the ear decompensates.

The tinnitus and fluctuant hearing loss may precede the attack of vertigo by days or even years and vice versa. We avoid the terms 'cochlear Ménière's disease', 'vestibular Ménière's disease' and 'monosymptomatic Ménière's disease', but prefer the terms 'hydrops of the pars cochlearis' and 'hydrops of the pars vestibularis', the term 'Ménière's disease' being reserved for the fully developed syndrome.

The most impressive feature of Ménière's disease is the acute episode of vertigo and hearing loss which is sometimes preceded by a sensation of fullness or pressure in the ear, and tinnitus. Nutritional, biochemical or mechanical changes in the inner ear are thought to be responsible for this sudden alteration in sensory function. The acuteness of the attack and the histological findings led Lawrence and McCabe (1959) and later Schuknecht *et al.* (1962) to postulate an episodic leakage of endolymph into the perilymphatic system as the cause of the symptoms. Escaping endolymph rich in potassium was proposed to have a toxic effect on the afferent neurons of the eighth cranial nerve. This interpretation was supported by Tasaki and Fernandez (1952), Dohlmann (1965) and Silverstein (1970). Their animal experiments proved that perfusion of the perilymphatic space with 'artificial' endolymph abolished the cochlear microphonics and produced severe nystagmus. This simple concept was readily accepted.

Despite some histological proof, the question whether endolymphatic membrane ruptures are artefacts remains unanswered. In the opinion of Jahnke (1977), one of my co-workers, the rupture hypothesis is questionable. Schuknecht and Seifi (1963) made ruptures in the cochlear duct in cats and thereby created permanent fistulae. They found that the biochemical and bioelectric properties of the cochlear duct a few millimetres distant from the fistula were maintained. This was confirmed by

Lawrence in 1965. Thus, only numerous ruptures or a very extensive rupture can explain the symptoms of a Ménière's attack.

Electron microscopic studies showed that the zonulae occludentes, the intercellular junctions surrounding the apical part of the cells in a belt- or band-like manner, are the main sealing elements of the endolymph–perilymph barrier. They therefore also influence the ion transport across the epithelial barrier. Jahnke (1977) postulates that 'the endolymphatic hydrops and the increased osmotic pressure of the endolymphatic hydrops destroys some of the intramembranous fibrils of the zonulae occludentes thereby disturbing their functions. This leads to leakage of the endolymph into the perilymph'. This may be true in other disorders of membrane metabolism, e.g. in endocrine disorders. Such a 'diffuse membrane leakage' may develop suddenly in cases where there is a disturbance in the microcirculation. Other authors also postulated that a sudden increase in potassium in the perilymph could have a toxic effect on the sensory and neural structures which are normally bathed in perilymph. In addition, the generation of a receptor potential is impaired by an accumulation of sodium ions or other electrolytes in the endolymph. The low-frequency hearing loss is associated with a functional disorder in the apex of the cochlea. This may be due to an extremely high ion exchange across the extended Reissner membrane so that the potassium ions diffuse directly from the scala vestibuli to scala tympani at the helicotrema. This does, however, not exclude mechanical factors (Tonndorf, 1968) as the cause of the low-frequency hearing loss.

This short discussion of the anatomy, histopathology and pathophysiology of ears with Ménière's disease might be helpful in deciding how to manage these patients.

Management

We certainly cannot alter the pneumatization of the temporal bone, the special location of the sac or the perisaccular fibrosis.

During the early stages of the disease, the elimination of the 'trigger' factor is often successful. The 'work-up' used in our department for every patient with unilateral deafness enables us to pin-point a possible trigger when the patient is seen for the first time. A carefully taken history gives additional information about stress, cigarette smoking, high salt intake, allergy and psychological problems. The latter seems to us to be more important than, for instance, House tends to believe (personal communication). If conservative treatment fails to control the vertiginous attacks, surgery is indicated.

The modification of Portmann's (1927) sac operation, namely opening the sac and inserting a triangular piece of silastic, is by no means a very successful procedure. It is rare to achieve a useful hearing gain, except in early cases with fluctuant hearing loss in the low-frequency range, which show hearing improvement after administration of glycerol. Elimination of vertiginous attacks is achieved in a fair percentage of cases. We therefore relieve the patient of the most distressing symptom by doing this rather small and safe procedure under local anaesthesia. The number of patients who require sectioning of the vestibular nerve via the middle cranial fossa or the translabyrinthine approaches is reduced by the sac operation.

An example of the role possibly played by *septic foci* on the function of the cochlea is illustrated by a patient who was admitted to our hospital with unilateral fluctuant hearing loss and an episode of vertigo and tinnitus of 1 year's duration. The work-up, including meatocysternography, was normal and medical treatment failed. Surgery for an opaque right maxillary sinus led to immediate and complete recovery of the fluctuant hearing loss, vertigo and tinnitus.

A patient with bilateral fluctuant hearing loss who had two episodes of sudden deafness on the right side suffered from spinning vertigo after extreme head movements. The removal of a right *cervical rib* resulted in full recovery of the hearing on that side. Fluctuant hearing loss on the left side and vertigo following head movements to the left was improved after the left cervical rib had been removed.

The cause of the sensory fluctuant hearing loss in this case was probably mechanical irritation of the sympathetic chain.

FLUCTUANT NEURAL (RETROCOCHLEAR) HEARING LOSS

Acoustic neuroma

Fluctuant hearing loss of neural origin is sometimes found in patients with small acoustic neuromas. These patients usually present with a slow progressive hearing loss. Some may present with sudden deafness which occasionally fully or partially recovers with conservative treatment. The fluctuant hearing loss may be a result of interference with cochlear blood supply due to the tumour affecting internal auditory artery flow. It may also be due to direct pressure on the nerve, or secondary to the marked increase in perilymph proteins.

Congenital cholesteatoma

As in patients with vestibular Schwannomas, we found a fluctuant hearing loss which progressed to a severe non-fluctuant hearing loss in one patient with congenital cholesteatoma. Full recovery of hearing occurred 4 months after the cholesteatoma was removed. The patient had been deaf for many years prior to surgery; this demonstrates the enormous potential of recovery of the eighth nerve.

Arachnoidal cysts

Arachnoidal cysts are another cause of fluctuant neural deafness. Surgery in three cases did not result in any improvement of hearing.

Multiple sclerosis

Fluctuant hearing loss of the neural type might also be due to multiple sclerosis. The demyelinating process is followed by glial replacement and eventual sclerotic plaque formation. Corresponding to the nature of the disease, the hearing loss does not follow consistent patterns. Frequently the hearing loss is of sudden onset, with a high incidence of spontaneous complete recovery. According to Citron *et al.* (1963), the recovery of speech discrimination lagged behind the recovery of pure tone thresholds.

Abnormalities of base of skull and the craniocervical region

Last but not least one should consider cochleo-vestibular disturbances related to abnormalities of the base of the skull and the craniocervical region. Platybasia, basilar impression and extension of the dens axis into the foramen magnum usually are inherited and only rarely acquired disorders. As the fully developed syndrome has symptoms and signs of brain stem compression and involvement of the cranial nerves VIII–XII, these patients are usually diagnosed and treated by neurologists and neurosurgeons.

Craniocervical dysplasia is of special importance to the otologist because otological symptoms and signs precede those of brain stem and other cranial nerve involvement. The diagnosis of craniocervical dysplasias can be readily made with the help of plain lateral skull X-rays or tomography. The most important feature is the relationship of the dens axis to different guide lines such as McGregor's or Chamberlain's line. The CAT scan is also very useful in demonstrating the relationship between the dens or the odontoid process and the medulla oblongata.

Gerlach (1954) and Unger, Ehrig and Eger (1973) described the occurrence of sensorineural hearing loss in patients with platybasia and Gerlach demonstrated a dramatic hearing improvement after neurosurgical enlargement of the posterior part of the foramen magnum.

According to the neurosurgical literature the incidence of vertigo, fluctuant hearing loss and tinnitus is 75% in these cases of 'basilar impression'.

My colleague Dr Elies, a neurosurgeon, found craniocervical dysplasia in 18.8% of 425 patients with vertigo, fluctuant hearing loss and tinnitus. The mean age in this group of 80 patients was 52 years; there was no special sex incidence (Elies and Plester, 1980). Most patients had unilateral, fluctuant, slowly progressive hearing loss in combination with unilateral tinnitus and suffered from vertigo which was symptomatically different from that of Ménière's disease, i.e. it was related to head movements and body flexion.

How can we explain the otological symptomatology from alterations of the bony structures in this region? In platybasia, disturbed circulation of cerebrospinal fluid may be responsible for the symptoms. The protruding odontoid process or dens axis may interfere with inner ear function by irritating the perivascular autonomic nerves of the vertebral and basilar arteries. This explanation is supported by the observation that vertigo and nystagmus occur during head movement. The high dens and the reactive fibrosis of the dura in adulthood lead to a progressive decrease in the calibre of the dura at the foramen magnum.

The incidence of craniocervical dysplasia in the normal population is 1:1500 (0.07%). In our series of 425 vertiginous patients with fluctuant hearing loss it was 18.8%. The otologist should therefore be aware of this syndrome; since it usually presents with otological symptoms, he is generally the first physician to see such a patient. As in acoustic neuromas, the treatment, including surgery, should be carried out by the neuro-otologist.

It has been my aim to show that fluctuant hearing loss is a symptom which can be due to a great number of factors. To elucidate the cause requires a thorough investigation, including otological, neurological and radiological examination. In the great majority of cases the inner ear is at fault, but we always have to look for trigger mechanisms elsewhere which have an adverse influence on the inner ear.

SUMMARY

Fluctuant hearing loss may have its genesis in the middle or inner ear, or in their central neural connections. Occasionally a fluctuating loss has its origins in combined middle and inner ear pathology and as a consequence both stable and non-stable components operate simultaneously. Reversal of the variable component is obviously possible. Middle ear effusion, the otomandibular syndrome and fistulae of the oval and round windows sometimes show such dual components. Endolymphatic hydrops and/or Ménière's disease provide the classical picture of fluctuating sensorineural deafness.

In a rather small percentage of cases acoustic neuroma demonstrates a hearing loss which is reversible. The same may apply to congenital cholesteatoma, arachnoid cysts, multiple sclerosis and abnormalities of the skull base and craniocervical region. The 'sudden deafness' syndrome often improves spontaneously and thus perhaps alludes to a vascular aetiology. Since the aetiologies of fluctuant deafness are legion their study requires, on occasion, a multidisciplinary approach.

References

Arenberg, I. K., Rask-Andersen, H., Wilbrand, H. and Stahle, J. (1977) The surgical anatomy of the endolymphatic sac. *Archives of Otolaryngology*, **103,** 1–11

Arnold, W. and Ganzer, U. (1980) Seromucotympanum and bone conduction. Proposed new classification of ear disease caused by Eustachian tube dysfunction. In *Physiology and Pathology of Eustachian Tube and Middle Ear* (International Symposium, Freiburg, 1977), pp. 71–78, p. 194. Georg Thieme Verlag

Citron, L., Dix, M., Hallpike, C. and Hood, J. (1963) A recent clinicopathological study of cochlear nerve degeneration resulting from tumor pressure and disseminated sclerosis, with particular reference to the finding of normal threshold sensitivity for pure tones. *Acta Otolaryngologica* (*Stockholm*), **56,** 330–337

Dohlmann, G. (1965) The mechanism of secretion and absorption of endolymph in the vestibular apparatus. *Acta Otolaryngologica (Stockholm)*, **59**, 275–288

Elies, W. and Plester, D. (1980) A differential diagnosis of Ménière's disease. *Archives of Otolaryngology*, **106**, 232–233

Gerlach, H. (1954) Die Beziehungen der Innenohrschwerhörigkeit zu den chronischen Liquorzirkulationsstörungen (mit besonderer Berücksichtigung der Schädelanomalien). *Acta Otolaryngologica (Stockholm)*, **4**, 324–335

Hlobil, H. (1979) Beeinflusst das Seromucotympanon die Sauerstoffversorgung des Innenohres? Eine klinisch-audiometrische Untersuchung. *Inaugural Dissertation*, University of Tübingen, Germany

Huizing, E. H. (1964) Pseudoperceptive deafness in tubotympanitis, sequelae of otitis media and otosclerosis. *Practica Oto-Rhino-Laryngologica (Basel)*, **26**, 225–226

Jahnke, K. (1977) Zur Pathogenese der akuten Symptome des Morbus Ménière. *Zeitschrift für Laryngologie und Rhinologie*, **56**, 402–406

Klockhoff, I. (1976) Diagnosis of Ménière's disease. *Archives of Oto-Rhino-Laryngology*, **212**(4), 309–314

Klockhoff, I. and Westerberg, C. E. (1973) A tonic tensor tympani phenomenon in man and its clinical significance. Excerpta Medica International Congress Series No. 176. World Congress of Otolaryngology, pp. 187–188 Amsterdam: Excerpta Medica

Lawrence, M. (1965) Fluid balance in the inner ear. *American Journal of Oto-Rhino-Laryngology*, **74**, 486

Lawrence, M. and McCabe, B. (1959) Inner ear mechanics and deafness. Special consideration of Ménière's syndrome. *Journal of the American Medical Association*, **1927** 171

Münker, G. (1980) The patulous Eustachian tube. In *Physiology and Pathology of Eustachian Tube and Middle Ear* (International Symposium, Freiburg, 1977). Stuttgart Georg Thieme Verlag

Pirker, C. (1976) Über Pneumatisationsverhältnisse des Schläfenbeins bei Morbus Ménière. *Inaugural Dissertation*, University of Tübingen, Germany

Plester, D. (1972) Surgery of endolymphatic hydrops. *Journal of the Oto-Laryngological Society of Australia*, **3**, 3

Portmann, G. (1927) Vertigo: surgical treatment by opening saccus endolymphaticus. *Archives of Otolaryngology*, **6**, 309

Schuknecht, H., Benites, J., Beekhuis, J., Igarashi, M., Singleton, C. and Ruedi, L. (1962) Pathology of sudden deafness. *Laryngoscope*, **72**, 1142–1157

Schuknecht, H. and Seifi, A. (1963) Experimental observations on the fluid physiology of the inner ear. *Annals of Otology, Rhinology and Laryngology*, **72**, 687

Shambaugh, G. (1975) Effect of endolymphatic sac decompression on fluctuant hearing loss. *Otolaryngological Clinics of North America*, **8**(2), 537–540

Silverstein, H. (1970) The effects of perfusing the perilymphatic space with artificial endolymph. *Annals of Otology, Rhinology and Laryngology*, **79**, 754

Tasaki, I. and Fernandez, C. (1952) Modification of cochlear microphonics and action potentials by KCl solution and direct current. *Journal of Neurophysiology*, **15**, 497–512

Tonndorf, J. (1968) Pathophysiology of the hearing loss of Ménière's disease. *Otolaryngological Clinics of North America*, **1**, 375

Unger, E., Ehrig, J. and Eger, H. (1973) Die basiläre Impression als Ursache kochleovestibulärer Störungen. *Zeitschrift für Laryngologie, Rhinologie und Otologie*, **52**, 114–120

13
Ototoxicity
John C. Ballantyne

Ototoxicity may be defined as damage by drugs to the cochlear and/or vestibular part of the inner ear. It has almost certainly existed for as long as drugs have been used, but scant attention was paid to it until the development of 'therapeutic agents of highly specific, permanent ototoxic effect' (Hawkins, 1967). These, of course, are the aminoglycoside antibiotics.

Any of these drugs may damage the cochlear or vestibular part of the labyrinth, or both, at least in experimentally induced changes in animals, but kanamycin, neomycin and vancomycin are particularly cochleotoxic, whereas gentamicin, streptomycin and tobramycin are particularly vestibulotoxic. Gentamicin and sissomicin can cause severe toxic damage to both parts.

There are considerable differences between species in their responses to aminoglycosides, but the reasons for these differences have yet to be explained.

No route of administration is exempt from danger, and ototoxic damage can be caused by topical application as well as by systemic administration, whether by injection or by ingestion.

Greater attention has been paid to the effects of the aminoglycosides than to those of the many other drugs which can be ototoxic, doubtless because in man the ototoxic effects of the former are almost always permanent and sometimes disastrous. This is not to say that the toxic effects of other drugs are always transient or reversible. Indeed, any or all of them have been reported to cause permanent damage on occasion, but some of the more important ones – notably the loop diuretics (frusemide/furosemide and ethacrynic acid), antiprotozoal agents (particularly quinine and chloroquine) and salicylates – are known more commonly to produce reversible effects.

The total list of drugs which may damage hearing or balance is a truly formidable one (Ballantyne, 1979) and, in addition to those already mentioned it includes: analeptics (including caffeine), anaesthetic agents (topical but not general), anticonvulsants, antidepressants, antidiabetic agents (including insulin), antiheparinizing and antihypertensive agents, anti-inflammatory drugs, contraceptives, cytotoxic agents, drugs used for the relief of cardiovascular conditions, sedatives and tranquillizers (including thalidomide).

Regrettably there is still much ignorance about the ototoxic effects of drugs, and the problem is compounded by the widespread use of proprietary names – especially for 'mixed' preparations – which give little or no idea of content.

ROUTES OF ACCESS TO THE INNER EAR

Drugs may be administered either systemically or topically: systemically by injection or ingestion; topically by application to any available surface or cavity, especially in the treatment of burns, in which there may be large surface areas for absorption.

When any drug is given systemically, or when one of the ototoxic antibiotics is applied topically to areas other than the ears themselves, it is carried to the labyrinthine fluids in the blood stream. It may be secreted into the perilymph from the vessels of the spiral ligament or directly into the endolymph from the stria vascularis (Hawkins, Beger and Aran, 1967); another possible route is from the vas spirale of the cochlea into the cortilymph.

When the aminoglycosides are applied topically to the middle ear (Spoendlin, 1966; Kohonen and Tarkkanen, 1969), they probably enter the perilymph by permeating the round window membrane; thence they may reach the organ of Corti by penetrating into the endolymphatic space from the scala vestibuli through Reissner's membrane.

These drugs are probably eliminated from the inner ear by resorption in the stria vascularis (Osteyn and Tyberghein, 1968) but, since the stria may itself be damaged by their toxic products (thus slowing still further the rate of resorption), they are eliminated more slowly from the labyrinthine fluids than from the blood. Hence their level remains higher and for a longer time in the inner ear than in the blood stream (Stupp and Rauch, 1965; Voldrich, 1965).

PHARMACOKINETICS

In 1967 Stupp *et al.* expressed the opinion that the ototoxic effects of the aminoglycoside antibiotics were related to their high concentration and prolonged presence in the labyrinthine fluids. They have shown, for example, that 24 hours after the administration of streptomycin the drug has been almost totally eliminated from the serum, whereas its concentration in the perilymph remains high.

In 1976 Federspil, Schützle and Tiesler investigated the ototoxic effects of gentamicin, tobramycin and amikacin. They estimated their concentrations in the serum, perilymph, cerebrospinal fluid and eye fluids over a period of 25 hours following subcutaneous injections of different doses and demonstrated that these drugs were retained for a long time in the inner ear fluids, the half-lives of gentamicin, tobramycin and amikacin in the perilymph being 12, 11 and 10 hours respectively. They too concluded that the ototoxic effect of the aminoglycoside antibiotics could best be explained by their concentrations in the inner ear fluids. Furthermore, they were able to demonstrate a linear relationship between the dosage of gentamicin and its concentration in the perilymph. They stated that in the guinea pig the level of ototoxicity of tobramycin is about half that of gentamicin.

However, more recently this concept has been challenged by Brummett *et al.* (1978), who found that although netilmicin had a longer half-life in perilymph than gentamicin, the former was nevertheless much less ototoxic than the latter.

Harpur (1982), in a study of the kinetics of ribostamycin in guinea pigs, has shown that after a *single dose* the half-life (15 hours) of ribostamycin in perilymph was much longer than its half-life (1 hour) in serum; at 12 hours there was a linear relationship between dose and perilymph concentration. However, after *multiple dosing* there was no evidence of any accumulation of the drug either in the serum or in the perilymph and there was no measurable retention of the drug in either fluid 2 weeks after the last of 14 daily injections. Indeed, after multiple dosing the drug appeared to be eliminated more rapidly. Harpur warns that the kinetics of aminoglycosides in the labyrinthine fluids and the relationship of kinetics to toxicity may be more complex than has previously been thought.

MECHANISM OF OTOTOXICITY

The exact mechanism by which certain drugs exert toxic effects on the inner ear is not known.

Hawkins (1973) has suggested that just as there is an effective blood–brain barrier so there may be a similar (but less effective) blood–ear barrier which may be capable of impeding the entrance of blood-borne substances into the inner ear fluids.

This 'haemato–labyrinthine barrier' may be bypassed, and the ototoxic process thereby greatly accelerated, by placing the drug directly into the middle ear (Spoendlin, 1966; Wersäll, Lundquist and Björkroth, 1969); permeation through the round window membrane will then exert an 'explosive' toxic effect on the neuro-epithelial structures of the inner ear.

The blood–ear barrier must depend on the integrity of the stria vascularis and spiral ligament whose microvasculature is primarily responsible for the elaboration of the labyrinthine fluids; there is evidence that the aminoglycosides damage these 'secretory' tissues.

Ototoxicity and renal status

The risk of ototoxicity is greatly increased by defective renal and, to a lesser extent, by defective hepatic function.

Since most of the ototoxic drugs are eliminated in the urine, impairment of renal function will permit high levels to develop in the plasma, and it has been emphasized (Ballantyne, 1970; Miszke, 1972) that patients with renal dysfunction are particularly susceptible to toxic effects.

Many of the ototoxic antibiotics are nephrotoxic, and the loop diuretics will rarely cause hearing loss save in patients with renal failure.

In this context there is special interest in the few cases of ototoxic damage which followed the use of the antiheparinizing agent hexadimethrine bromide (Ransome *et al.*, 1966) now no longer used. There are certain close resemblances between the glomerular tufts of the kidneys and the structure of the stria vascularis, and the drug is known to be nephrotoxic in high doses. Haller *et al.* (1962) described a 'constriction of the capillaries within the glomerular tufts', and it is possible that this drug may act in a similar way upon the microvasculature of the cochlea.

Ototoxic synergism

There is much anecdotal (and some experimental) evidence that the risk of toxic damage from any potentially ototoxic drug is considerably augmented by previous treatment with the same or other ototoxic agents, e.g. antimalarial drugs (Nilges and Northern, 1971), diuretics (West, Brummett and Himes, 1973) or ototoxic antibiotics (Frost, Hawkins and Daly, 1960) – or even by previous exposure to noise (Darrouzet and de Lima Sobrinho, 1963).

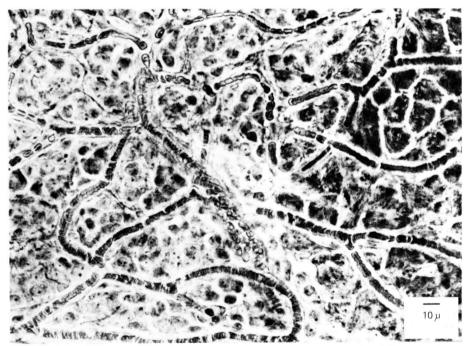

Figure 13.1 Atrophy of stria vascularis, showing normal vessels to the right with 'ghosts' of capillaries to the left. (By courtesy of Dr Joseph E. Hawkins, Jr, Kresge Hearing Research Institute, Ann Arbor, Michigan, USA)

HISTOPATHOLOGY OF OTOTOXICITY

The aminoglycoside antibiotics

Johnsson and Hawkins (1972) emphasized that although the hair cells and first-order neurons of the eighth cranial nerve have been generally regarded as the primary sites of ototoxic damage, several forms of sensorineural hearing loss are associated with vascular changes in the cochlea, and that these changes often precede, and may be an important cause of, degenerative changes in the hair cells.

Severe strial atrophy was seen in cats which had received large doses of neomycin. This was most marked in the basal turn, where only empty remnants ('ghosts') of capillaries and intervascular strands (*Figure 13.1*) remained.

Johnsson and Hawkins (1972) studied other changes in the microvasculature of guinea pigs treated with gentamicin and were able to demonstrate (in the spiral ligament and external sulcus) destruction of the pericapillary spaces – specialized spaces which surround the capillary networks in this region and which appear to be characteristic of vessels actively engaged in filtration and/or reabsorption of fluid.

The histopathological changes which occur in the sensory epithelia of the labyrinth have been extensively studied in animals by light and phase-contrast microscopy, and by electron microscopy and scanning electron microscopy.

Cochleotoxicity

For many years, the surface preparation technique of Engström (1951) has formed the basis of many animal studies, notably in guinea pigs, in which the hair cells form a remarkably constant and regular pattern (*Figure 13.2*). It is a quick and relatively simple method which is particularly well suited to the study of hair cell damage.

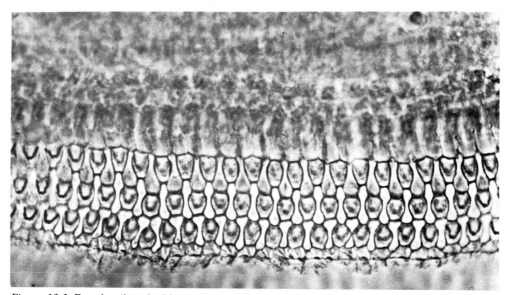

Figure 13.2 Regular 'interlocking' pattern of outer hair cells in the guinea pig's normal cochlea. (By courtesy of Professor Hans Engström, Academic Hospital, Uppsala, Sweden)

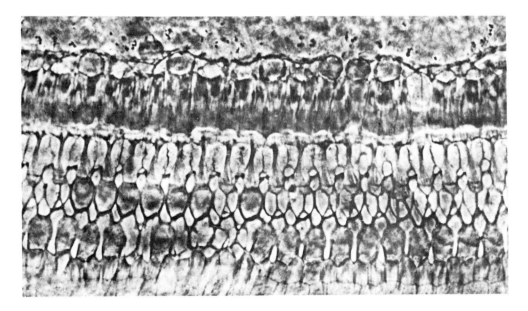

Figure 13.3 Guinea pig's cochlea damaged by kanamycin. 'Collapse figures' replace all the hair cells in the first row of outer hair cells; there are also many in the second row, and a few in the third row. (By courtesy of Professor Hans Engström, Academic Hospital, Uppsala, Sweden)

The changes seen in cases of cochlear toxicity have been remarkably consistent. At first there is distortion of the normal W-pattern of the sterocilia surmounting the outer hair cells (these changes are particularly well seen in scanning electron microscopy). With increasing damage, the hairs are entirely lost and the whole cell may disappear, leaving a 'collapse body' or 'phalangeal scar' (*Figure 13.3*).

The outer hair cells of the basal turn are affected first, the damage later progressing towards the apex; the inner hair cells, which are affected much later, degenerate in the opposite direction.

The extent of damage to the hair cells can be conveniently and graphically recorded in a cochlear cytogram or 'cochleogram' (*Figure 13.4*).

Kanamycin 400 mg/kg body weight
for 8 days, sacrificed 14 days later.
2 1/2 Coils from base.

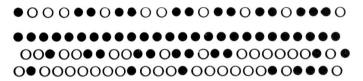

Figure 13.4 'Cochlear cytogram' of a guinea pig's cochlea damaged by kanamycin. (○) Normal hair cell; (●) degenerated hair cell (By courtesy of Professor Hans Engström, Academic Hospital, Uppsala, Sweden

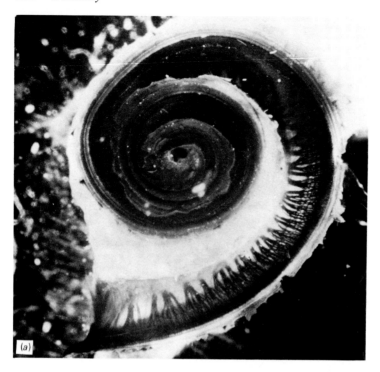

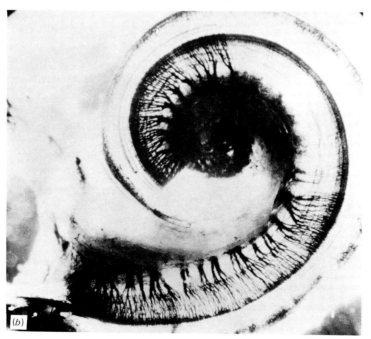

Figure 13.5 Cochlear nerve fibres of the guinea pig: (*a*) normal fibres; (*b*), degenerated fibres (pale areas) corresponding with the areas of damage to the hair cells. (By courtesy of Professor Hans Engström, Academic Hospital, Uppsala, Sweden)

Friedmann, Dadswell and Bird (1966) produced the first electron microscopic study of cochlear changes induced by neomycin and confirmed that damage to the organ of Corti in guinea pigs was most pronounced in the basal coil. Marked degeneration of the mitochondria was demonstrated in both outer and inner hair cells.

The results of animal experiments have been amply confirmed in microscopic examinations of human temporal bones and, with kanamycin, the findings in human ears have been identical with those of experimentally induced lesions in animals (Benitez, Schuknecht and Brandenburg, 1962; Jørgensen and Schmidt, 1962; Matz, Wallace and Ward, 1965).

Degeneration of the nerve fibres (*Figure 13.5*) occurs secondarily to degeneration of the sensory epithelia but, even with total loss of all hair cells, there is usually survival of 5–10% of the neurons (Spoendlin, 1974).

Vestibulotoxicity

In an electron microscopic study of the ototoxicity of gentamicin, Wersäll and Lundquist (1967) expressed the view that the primary site of damage to the vestibular labyrinth was in the sensory cells.

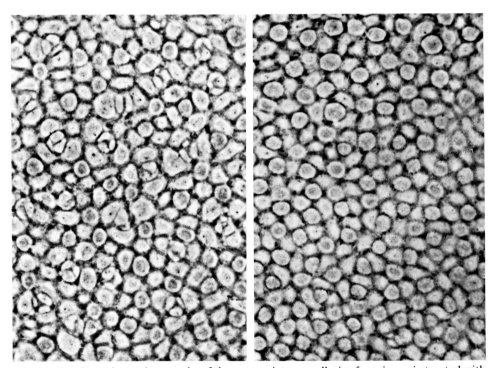

Figure 13.6 Two photomicrographs of the same crista ampullaris of a guinea pig treated with kanamycin, showing a high proportion of degenerated sensory cells ('collapse figures') in the central areas (left) and normal sensory epithelium in the peripheral areas (right). (By courtesy of Dr Henrik H. Lindeman, Ullevål Hospital, Oslo, Norway)

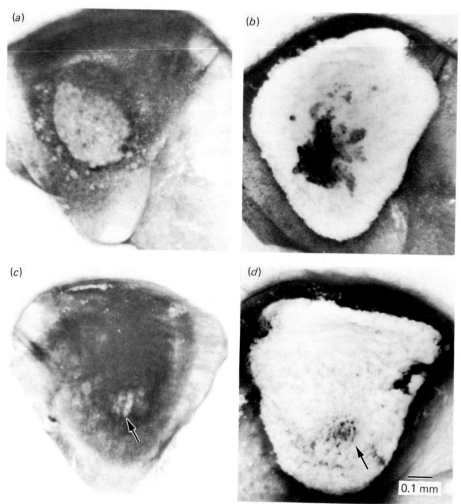

Figure 13.7 Utricular maculae from two different animals. The otoconial membranes (right) have been dissected away to show the corresponding epithelial defects (left). Large defects are seen in (*a*) and (*b*) 20 days after 'treatment' with streptomycin; (*c*) and (*d*) show smaller lesions (arrows) close to the posterior tip of the macula, 6 days after 'treatment' (By courtesy of Dr Lars-Göran Johnsson, Kresge Hearing Research Institute, Ann Arbor, Michigan, USA

In his studies on the sensory region, Lindeman (1969a, 1969b) investigated the effects of streptomycin and kanamycin on the vestibular epithelia and found clear regional differences in vulnerability. After parenteral administration of kanamycin, he noted a high proportion of degenerated cells in the central areas of the ampullary cristae, with normal epithelia in the peripheral areas (*Figure 13.6*).

These cristae of the semicircular canals were more vulnerable than the maculae, and the utricular macula was more vulnerable than the saccular macula. Toyoda *et al.* (1977) have demonstrated similar changes in guinea pigs which had received kanamycin.

Johnsson *et al.* (1980) recently made a study of streptomycin-induced defects in the otoconial membrane. A circumscribed loss of otoconia was seen in the posterior half of the macula utriculi (*Figure 13.7*), and examination with the scanning electron microscope of the margins of these defects showed that some of the otoconia were in the process of degenerating: their surfaces were uneven, with pitting and small grooves running longitudinally; in advanced stages of degeneration, the otoconia were hollowed out, leaving a shell.

In every specimen in which these otoconial changes were present, epithelial defects were found which corresponded both in size and in location to a defect in the otoconial layer.

The vestibular secretory tissues which correspond to the stria vascularis in the cochlea are the 'dark cells', which appear on the slopes of the ampullary cristae; Hawkins and Preston (1975) have demonstrated shrinkage and vacuolization of these cells in experimental animals after streptomycin and gentamicin.

Diuretics

Ethacrynic acid and frusemide, although differing in chemical structure, have similar actions on the renal tubules, where they inhibit reabsorption of sodium and water in the proximal portion of the loop of Henle (Hawkins, 1976), and it is interesting that the main histopathological change in the inner ear has been one of strial atrophy, most marked in the basal turn of the cochlea.

In 1970 Quick and Duvall demonstrated strial damage in guinea pigs, and two years later Johnsson and Hawkins (1972) confirmed this in cats. Swollen osmiophilic cells were clumped around the capillaries, and there were light bare zones between the capillary loops and also numerous small vacuoles in the spiral ligament.

Arnold, Nadol and Weidaner (1981) have reported the interesting case of a patient who suffered from sudden deafness and ataxia after the administration of both frusemide and ethacrynic acid. Although there was no actual loss of hair cells or supporting cells, there were marked changes in the stria vascularis of the cochlea and in the 'dark cell' areas of the vestibular labyrinth.

Antiprotozoal agents and salicylates

The effects of both antiprotozoal agents (quinine and chloroquine) and salicylates are probably brought about by vasoconstriction of the small vessels of the cochlear microvasculature (Hawkins, Beger and Aran, 1967).

In 1964 Matz and Naunton reported complete absence of hair cells and loss of many supporting cells in the organ of Corti in the offspring of a mother to whom chloroquine had been administered during the first three months of her pregnancy.

Three years later McKinna (1967) reported two cases of congenital deafness in infants whose mothers had taken high prenatal doses of quinine; degenerative changes were found in the spiral ganglion cells.

CLINICAL FEATURES OF OTOTOXICITY

Tinnitus

Tinnitus is often the first symptom of cochleotoxic damage. It is associated particularly with salicylates and antiprotozoal agents, and with both these groups of drugs it is usually reversible.

High-pitched tinnitus is often the earliest symptom of aminoglycoside cochleo-toxicity and is usually present before there is any subjective hearing loss (Ballan-tyne, 1976). Its persistent presence is always suggestive of impending deafness, and an audiogram should be done as soon as possible.

Deafness

The hearing loss of aminoglycoside ototoxicity is always sensorineural in nature and, as one would expect from the cochlear cytogram, it affects mainly and progressively the high frequencies at first (*Figure 13.8*). Most commonly it follows parenteral administration, but it may also follow oral (Ballantyne, 1970) or topical application.

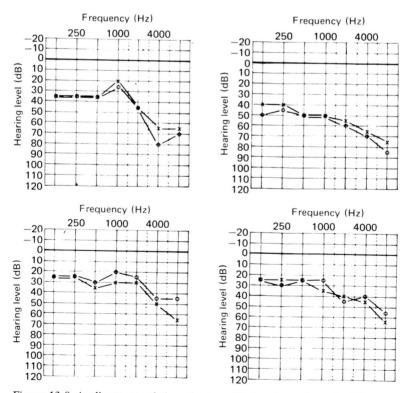

Figure 13.8 Audiograms of 4 patients suffering from hepatic failure treated with oral neomycin. (○—○) Right air conduction; (×—×) left air conduction. (Patients of Professor Sheila Sherlock, Royal Free Hospital, London, UK)

Not infrequently the hearing loss may appear after a long latent period; and, indeed, it may sometimes be first noticed after the drug has been discontinued and may even progress thereafter – sometimes for weeks or months. It is irreversible.

There appears to be some familial predisposition to ototoxic deafness (Miszke, 1972), and, even with ordinary doses, dangerous concentrations of aminoglycosides may appear in the serum in the very young and very old. These drugs may also cross the placental barrier in concentrations sufficiently high to damage the fetal ear.

Hearing loss due to diuretics usually follows intravenous injection and it occurs especially in uraemic patients; it is usually immediate in onset but most often

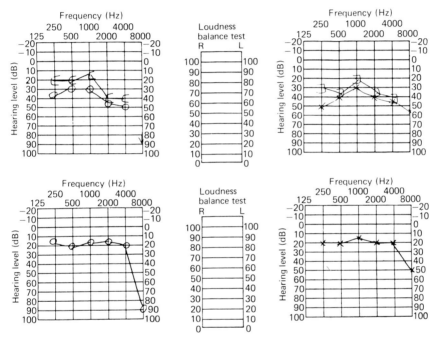

Figure 13.9 Audiograms of a patient with hepatic failure treated with bromocriptine, showing hearing after treatment with a 'standard' dose of bromocriptine (top) and improvement in hearing 6 months after reduction of dosage (bottom). (o—o) Right air conduction; ([—[) right bone conduction; (×—×) left air conduction; (]—]) left bone conduction. (Patient of Dr Marsha Morgan, Royal Free Hospital, London, UK

transient. So too is the deafness caused by salicylates, although in both instances the loss may be permanent; the same applies to antiprotozoal agents.

There are, of course, many other drugs which have been reported to cause occasional deafness: thalidomide, now fortunately no longer available, could cause cochlear lesions in addition to the more common congenital anomalies of the outer and middle ears (Livingstone, 1965); practolol appears to be unique amongst β-blocking agents in its ability to cause deafness, often with a mixture of sensorineural loss and a conductive loss due to serous otitis media. Characteristic-ally the deafness was noticed months or even years after the appearance of other side-effects, notably a skin rash and dry eyes (McNab Jones *et al.*, 1977). Cytotoxic agents, notably nitrogen mustard (Schuknecht, 1964; Cummings, 1968) and Cisplatin (*cis*-platinum) (Johnson, 1982; Chapman, 1982), may also damage the hearing.

Another interesting drug, previously unreported, is bromocriptine, which has been used successfully in a very limited number of patients with hepatic failure. It was given to patients who developed portosystemic encephalopathy, the complication of liver disease for which neomycin has been widely used in the past (Morgan, 1981). A similar type of hearing loss, affecting mainly the high tones, was noted, but differing from neomycin-induced deafness in that it appears to be reversible (*Figure 13.9*) with reduction of dosage.

Ataxia and vertigo

Streptomycin and gentamicin are predominantly vestibulotoxic.

The onset of dizziness may be sudden or gradual, usually starting with slight dysequilibrium in the dark or on sudden movement. Ataxia may also occur, with a tendency to fall, and there may be visual difficulties in walking. This 'bobbing oscillopsia' has been studied by Ramsden (1982) in 15 patients who had suffered severe labyrinthine damage from gentamicin. None of the patients had severe vertigo but all of them complained of a vertical bouncing of their surroundings, occurring with each step during walking.

The caloric responses are usually absent or grossly reduced, as is the horizontal nystagmus produced by rotation.

PREVENTION OF OTOTOXIC DAMAGE

The ototoxic effects of certain drugs are becoming increasingly well known, and there is a constant search for equally effective but less toxic alternatives. If such alternatives are available they should, of course, be used in preference to those of high toxicity. There is hope, for example, that some of the newer broad-spectrum cephalosporins and penicillins may one day replace the aminoglycosides, at least in some instances (Noone, 1982).

Unfortunately, however, that happy state has not yet been reached and it must be recognized that no drug is *absolutely* safe. In the meantime, therefore, it will be necessary to rely on the undoubted efficacy of such drugs as gentamicin in life-threatening sepsis and septicaemia, especially when associated with coliform organisms, staphylococci and *Ps. aeruginosa*.

When any of the aminoglycosides are prescribed, it is important to monitor the dosage effectively with serum assays; it has been found that trough levels are more accurate indicators of toxicity than peak concentrations (Noone, 1982).

In animal experimental work, the extent of damage observed in the labyrinth is almost always dose-related, but in humans the relationship of ototoxic damage to dosage is erratic (Ballantyne, 1970); not least amongst the various factors responsible for this discrepancy is the renal status of the patient.

Mawer *et al.* (1974) developed a computer programme from which they have constructed 'nomograms' for the calculation of kanamycin and gentamicin dosages (*Figure 13.10*), but 'wild variations in blood levels . . . may occur in renal impairment despite "accurate calculations"' (Quick, 1973).

Attempts to reduce the toxicity of certain drugs by the simultaneous use of others have so far been unsuccessful.

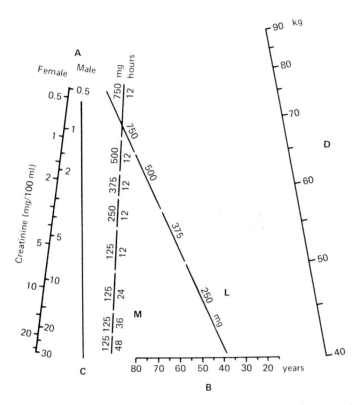

Figure 13.10 'Nomogram' for kanamycin dosage. A point is made on line A in accordance with sex and creatinine level; this point is joined by a straight line to another on line B, according to the patient's age. The point where this line crosses line C is then joined to a point on line D which indicates the patient's weight. This new line crosses lines L and M: the point at which it crosses line L indicates the initial 'loading' dose; the point at which it crosses line M indicates the 12-hourly maintenance dose. (Modified from Mawer *et al.*, 1974)

It therefore behoves the prescribing doctor to limit the prescription of ototoxic drugs to cases in which there is no effective alternative, especially in cases of renal or hepatic failure, in pregnant women and in the very young or the very old (Ballantyne, 1976). Extra caution should be exercised in patients who have previously been treated with any potentially ototoxic agent, in those who have been exposed to much noise and in those with a known incidence of ototoxicity in the family (Ballantyne, 1973).

Topical preparations should be applied with great care, especially to large surface areas, as in extensive burns. Despite the great toxicity of some aminoglycosides when applied directly to the middle ears of experimental animals, there are few reports of ototoxicity from the widespread use of drops in clinical practice. All patients receiving ototoxic drugs should be encouraged to report the onset of symptoms, however slight, of tinnitus, hearing loss, dizziness or ataxia; regular audiometric checks are recommended.

THE CLINICAL MANAGEMENT OF OTOTOXICITY

Although there have been reports of spontaneous recovery of hearing in cases of ototoxic deafness there is as yet no effective treatment for ototoxicity once it is established.

Cochleotoxicity

Ideally, serial audiograms should be begun before treatment is instituted and continued at regular intervals; if at all feasible, the drug should be withdrawn immediately any signs of hearing loss develop. If the loss warrants it, a hearing aid should be issued and rehabilitation begun.

Fortunately the hearing loss is not always severe, but some of the most profound losses recorded have followed the topical application of ototoxic antibiotics to extensive burned areas. It is of considerable interest that of the first 110 profoundly deaf patients implanted with single electrode cochlear implants (House *et al.*, 1981), 16% had been deafened by ototoxic antibiotics, some of them applied topically (Ballantyne, Evans and Morrison, 1978).

Vestibulotoxicity

Patients with vestibular symptoms may be helped by a graduated (Cooksey's) system of exercises originally designed for patients suffering from dysequilibrium after head injuries, and later used widely for those suffering from vertigo after the fenestration operation (Dix, 1980).

Cinnarizine has been found to be useful as a labyrinthine sedative (Oosterveld, 1980).

CONCLUSIONS

The last four decades have witnessed a veritable explosion of therapeutic possibilities. Many thousands of lives have been saved, but sometimes the cost of survival has been high; and ototoxicity is one the prices that has had to be paid.

No doubt ototoxicity will continue to exist, as it has probably existed from the earliest use of drugs. Absolute safety does not exist in medicine; but with the development of new and safer drugs, with improved techniques of preclinical tests and with more watchful monitoring for potentially toxic reactions, it is to be hoped that the incidence and severity of deafness and dizziness due to drugs will diminish.

References

Arnold, W., Nadol, J. B., Jr and Weidaner, H. (1981) Ultrastructural histopathology in a case of human ototoxicity due to loop diuretics. *Acta Otolaryngologica (Stockholm)*, **91**, 399–414

Ballantyne, J. C. (1970) Iatrogenic deafness. *Journal of Laryngology and Otology*, **84**, 967–1000

Ballantyne, J. C. (1973) Ototoxicity. A clinical review. *Audiology*, **12**, 325–336

Ballantyne, J. C. (1976) Ototoxic drugs. In *Scientific Foundations of Otolaryngology*, edited by R. Hinchcliffe and D. F. N. Harrison, pp. 849–862. London: William Heinemann Medical Books Ltd

Ballantyne, J. C. (1979) Ototoxicity. In *Diseases of the Ear, Nose and Throat*, edited by J. C. Ballantyne and J. Groves, Vol. 2, pp. 671–682. London: Butterworths

Ballantyne, J. C., Evans, E. F. and Morrison, A. W. (1978) Electrical auditory stimulation in the management of profound hearing loss. *Journal of Laryngology and Otology*, Suppl. 1, 1–117

Benitez, J. T., Schuknecht, H. F. and Brandenburg, J. H. (1962) Pathologic changes in human ear after kanamycin. *Archives of Otolaryngology*, **75**, 192–197

Brummett, R. E., Fox, K. E., Brown, R. T. and Himes, D. L. (1978) Comparative ototoxic liability of netilmicin and gentamicin. *Archives of Otolaryngology*, **104**, 579–584

Chapman, P. (1982) Rapid-onset *cis*-platinum therapy: case reports and literature review. *Journal of Laryngology and Otology* (in press)

Cummings, C. W. (1968) Experimental observations on the ototoxicity of nitrogen mustard. *Laryngoscope*, **78**, 530–538

Darrouzet, J. and de Lima Sobrinho, J. (1963) The internal ear, kanamycin and acoustic trauma. Experimental study. *Révue de Laryngologie, Otologie et Rhinologie*, **83**, 781–806

Dix, M. R. (1980) Head exercises in the treatment of vertigo. In *Cinnarizine and the Vertiginous Syndrome* (No. 33 of Royal Society of Medicine International Congress and Symposium Series), edited by G. Towse, pp. 23–28. London: Academic Press, Grune and Stratton

Engström, H. (1951) Microscopic anatomy of the inner ear. *Acta Otolaryngologica (Stockholm)*, **40**, 5–22

Federspil, P., Schützle, W. and Tiesler, E. (1976) Pharmacokinetics and ototoxicity of gentamicin, tobramycin and amikacin. *Journal of Infectious Diseases*, **134**, S200–S205

Friedmann, I., Dadswell, J. V. and Bird, E. S. (1966) Electron-microscope studies of the neuro-epithelium of the inner ear in guinea-pigs treated with neomycin. *Journal of Pathology and Bacteriology*, **92**, 415–422

Frost, J. O., Hawkins, J. E., Jr and Daly, J. F. (1960) Kanamycin: ototoxicity. *American Review of Respiratory Diseases*, **82**, 23–30

Haller, J. A., Jr, Ransdell, H. J., Jr, Stowens, D. and Rubel, W. F. (1962) Renal toxicity of Polybrene in open-heart surgery. *Journal of Thoracic and Cardiovascular Surgery*, **44**, 486–493

Harpur, E. S. (1982) Kinetics of drugs in perilymph in relation to toxicity. *British Journal of Audiology* (in press)

Hawkins, J. E., Jr (1967) Iatrogenic toxic deafness in children. In *Deafness in Children*, edited by F. McConnell and P. H. Ward, pp. 156–168. Nashville: Vanderbilt University Press

Hawkins, J. E., Jr (1973) Ototoxic mechanisms: a working hypothesis. *Audiology*, **12**, 383–393

Hawkins, J. E., Jr (1976) Drug ototoxicity. In *Handbook of Sensory Physiology*, Vol. 5, pp. 707–748. Berlin and Heidelberg: Springer-Verlag

Hawkins, J. E., Jr, Beger, V. and Aran, J.-M. (1967) Antibiotic insults to Corti's organ. In *Sensory Hearing Processes and Disorders*, edited by A. B. Graham, pp. 411–425. Boston: Little, Brown and Company

Hawkins, J. E., Jr and Preston, J. E. (1975) Vestibular ototoxicity. In *The Vestibular System*, edited by R. F. Naunton, pp. 321–349. New York: Academic Press

House, W. F., Berliner, K. I., Eisenberg, L. S., Edgerton, B. J. and Thielemeir, M. A. (1981) The cochlear implant: 1980 update. *Acta Otolaryngologica (Stockholm)*, **91**, 457–462

Johnson, T. F. (1982) Ototoxicity of *cis*-platinum in patients. *British Journal of Audiology* (in press)

Johnsson, L.-G. and Hawkins, J. E., Jr (1972) Strial atrophy in clinical and experimental deafness. *Laryngoscope*, **83**, 1105–1125

Johnsson, L.-G., Wright, C. G., Preston, R. E. and Henry, P. J. (1980) Streptomycin-induced defects of the otoconial membrane. *Acta Otolaryngologica (Stockholm)*, **89**, 401–406

Jørgensen, M. B. and Schmidt, M. R. (1962) The ototoxic effect of kanamycin. *Acta Otolaryngologica (Stockholm)*, **55**, 537–544

Kohonen, A. and Tarkkanen, J. (1969) Cochlear damage from ototoxic antibiotics by intratympanic application. *Acta Otolaryngologica (Stockholm)*, **68**, 90–97

Lindeman, H. (1969a) Regional differences in structure of the vestibular sensory regions. *Journal of Laryngology and Otology*, **83**, 1–17

Lindeman, H. (1969b) Regional differences in sensitivity of the vestibular sensory epithelia to ototoxic antibiotics. *Acta Otolaryngologica (Stockholm)*, **67**, 177–189

Livingstone, G. (1965) Congenital ear abnormalities due to thalidomide. *Proceedings of the Royal Society of Medicine*, **58**, 493–497

McKinna, A. J. (1967) Quinine induced hypoplasia of the optic nerve. *Canadian Journal of Ophthalmology*, **1**, 261–266

McNab Jones, R. F., Hammond, V. T., Wright, D. and Ballantyne, J. C. (1977) Practolol and deafness. *Journal of Laryngology and Otology*, **91**, 963–972

Matz, G. J. and Naunton, R. F. (1964) Ototoxicity of chloroquine. *Archives of Otolaryngology*, **88**, 370–372

Matz, G. J., Wallace, T. H. and Ward, P. H. (1965) The ototoxicity of kanamycin. A comparative histopathological study. *Laryngoscope*, **75**, 1690–1698

Mawer, G. E., Ahmad, R., Dobbs, S. M., McGouch, J. G., Lucas, S. B. and Tooth, J. A. (1974) Experience with a gentamicin nomogram. *Postgraduate Medical Journal*, **50** (Suppl. 7), 31–32

Miszke, A. (1972) Obserwacje nad wystepowaniem i ustepowaniem zaburzeń widenzia w przebiegu uszkodzén blednikớw streptomycyna. *Folia med Cracov*, **14**, 29–38

Morgan, M. Y. (1981) Bromocriptine in the treatment of chronic encephalopathy and its effects on the handling of alcohol by control subjects and alcoholics. *Research and Clinical Forums*, **3**(1), 39–47

Nilges, T. C. and Northern, J. L. (1971) Iatrogenic ototoxic hearing loss. *Annals of Surgery*, **173**, 281–289

Noone, P. (1982) Clinical use of aminoglycosides. *British Journal of Audiology* (in press)

Oosterveld, W. J. (1980) Cinnarizine in the vertiginous syndrome. In *Cinnarizine and the Vertiginous Syndrome* (No. 33 of Royal Society of Medicine International Congress and Symposium Series), edited by G. Towse, pp. 29–37. London: Academic Press, Grune and Stratton

Osteyn, F. and Tyberghein, J. (1968) Influence of some streptomyces antibiotics on the inner ear of the guinea pig. *Acta Otolaryngologica* (*Stockholm*), Suppl. 234, 5–91

Quick, C. A. (1973) Chemical and drug effects on the inner ear. In *Otolaryngology*, edited by M. M. Paparella and D. D. Shumrick, Vol. 2, pp. 397–406. Philadelphia: W. B. Saunders

Quick, C. A. and Duvall, A. J. (1970) Early changes in the cochlear duct from ethacrynic acid: an electronmicroscopic evaluation. *Laryngoscope*, **80**, 954–965

Ramsden, R. T. (1982) Bobbing oscillopsia from gentamicin toxicity. *British Journal of Audiology* (in press)

Ransome, J., Ballantyne, J. C., Shaldon, S., Bosher, K. and Hallpike, C. S. (1966) Perceptive deafness in subjects with renal failure treated with haemodialysis and Polybrene. *Journal of Laryngology and Otology*, **80**, 651–677

Schuknecht, H. F. (1964) The pathology of several disorders of the inner ear which cause vertigo. *Southern Medical Journal*, **57**, 1161–1167

Spoendlin, H. (1966) Zur Ototoxizität des Streptomyzins. *Practica Oto-rhino-laryngologica* (*Basel*), **28**, 305–322

Spoendlin, H. (1974) Neuroanatomy of the cochlea. In *Electrical Stimulation of the Acoustic Nerve in Man*, edited by M. M. Merzenich, R. A. Schindler and F. A. Sooy, pp. 7–23. San Francisco: Velo-Bind, Inc.

Stupp, H. F. and Rauch, S. (1965) Diskussion zu den Referaten und zu den Vorträgen. *Archiv für Ohren-, Nasen- und Kehlkopfkunde*, **185**, 500–501

Stupp, H. F., Rauch, S., Sous, H., Brun, J. P. and Lagler, F. (1967) Kanamycin dosage and levels in ear and other organs. *Archives of Otolaryngology*, **86,** 515–521

Toyoda, Y., Saito, H., Matsuoka, H., Takenaka, H., Oshima, W. and Mizukoshi, O. (1977) Quantitative analysis of kanamycin ototoxicity. *Acta Otolaryngologica (Stockholm)*, **84,** 202–217

Voldrich, L. (1965) The kinetics of streptomycin, kanamycin and neomycin in the inner ear. *Acta Otolaryngologica (Stockholm)*, **60,** 243–248

Wersäll, J. and Lundquist, P.-G. (1967) The ototoxic effect of gentamicin: an electron microscopic study. In *Gentamicin: First International Symposium*, pp. 24–46. Essex: Chenie Ag

Wersäll, J., Lundquist, P.-G. and Björkroth, B. (1969) Ototoxicity of gentamicin. *Journal of Infectious Diseases*, **119,** 410–416

West, B. A., Brummett, R. E. and Himes, D. L. (1973) Interaction of kanamycin and ethacrynic acid. *Archives of Otolaryngology*, **98,** 32–37

Index

252   *Index*